The ECG in practice

The ECG in practice

John Hampton DM, MA, DPhil, FRCP
Professor of Cardiology,
University of Nottingham,
Nottingham, UK

Churchill Livingstone

EDINBURGH LONDON MELBOURNE AND NEW YORK 1986

CHURCHILL LIVINGSTONE
Medical Division of Longman Group UK Limited

Distributed in the United States of America by Churchill Livingstone
Inc., 1560 Broadway, New York, N. Y. 10036, and by associated
companies, branches and representatives throughout the world.

First published 1986
  Reprinted 1987
  Reprinted 1988

ISBN 0 443 03324 2

British Library Cataloguing in Publication Data
Hampton, John R.
   The ECG in practice.
   1. Electrocardiography
   I. Title
   616.1'207547   RC683.5.E5

Library of Congress Cataloging in Publication Data
Hampton, John R.
   The ECG in practice.
   A companion v. to: The ECG made easy.
   1. Electrocardiography. 2. Heart — Disease —
Diagnosis. I. Hampton, John R. ECG made easy.
II. Title. [DNLM: 1. Electrocardiography.
WG 140 H232ea]
RC683.5.E5H3   1985   Suppl.   616.1'207547   85-26943

Produced by Longman Singapore Publishers (Pte) Ltd.
Printed in Singapore.

Preface

This book assumes the level of knowledge about the ECG that is contained in *The ECG Made Easy,* to which this is a companion volume. The principles underlying *The ECG Made Easy* are that the ECG is easy to understand, and that its abnormalities are amendable to reason. Both the normal ECG and the typical examples of abnormal ECGs are indeed easy to interpret, but the ECG sometimes appears more difficult than it really is because of the variations that can occur both in the normal record and in the abnormal ECGs that are associated with various diseases. This book therefore goes beyond the typical ECGs and attempts to describe the variations that are seen in health and disease.

The second purpose of this book is to demonstrate that an ECG should always be interpreted in the light of the individual subject from whom it was recorded. Recording and interpreting the ECG is, in fact, an extension of taking the clinical history and performing a physical examination. The ECG is not an end in itself, but is part of the process of diagnosis and management of an individual patient, so this book approaches the ECG from the clinical standpoint of the different symptoms of cardiovascular disease. To emphasise the secondary role of the ECG in diagnosis each chapter begins with a brief consideration of how the history and physical examination can be used to make, or at least suspect, a diagnosis so that the ECG can be used in the most intelligent and profitable way.

There is no point in recording an ECG unless you know what to do with the result, so at the end of each chapter there is a brief section outlining the action that should follow the identification of ECG abnormalities.

One of the fascinating things about the ECG is the amount of information it provides about the normal and pathological physiology of the heart. Knowing about this is by no means essential for making use of the ECG, but it certainly helps to understand it. Because many people will make good use of the ECG without ever wanting to know about its physiological basis, the description of this is placed in the final chapter which can be read or ignored according to the readers' interests and temperament.

I am grateful to many colleagues who helped me to find the ECGs that are included in this book, and I am particularly grateful to Mr G. Lyth for preparing the illustrations.

Nottingham, 1986   J.H.

Contents

Chapter 1
The ECG in healthy people

History and examination

For the purposes of this chapter we shall assume that the subject is asymptomatic, and that physical examination has revealed no abormalities. We need to consider the range of normality in the ECG, but of course we cannot escape from the fact that not all disease causes symptoms or abnormal physical signs, and a subject who appears healthy may not be so. In particular, individuals who present for 'screening' may well have symptoms about which they have not consulted a doctor, so it cannot be assumed that an ECG obtained through a screening programme has come from a healthy subject.

The range of normality of the ECG is therefore debatable; we have to consider the variations in the ECG that we can expect to find in completely healthy people, and then we can think about the significance of more marked abnormalities.

Acceptable variations in the normal ECG

The normal cardiac rhythm

Sinus rhythm is the only normal sustained rhythm. In young people the R-R interval is reduced (that is, the heart rate is increased) by inspiration and this is called sinus arrhythmia. When sinus arrhythmia is marked it may mimic an atrial arrhythmia. However, in sinus arrhythmia each P–QRS–T complex is normal, and it is only the interval between them that changes.

SINUS ARRHYTHMIA

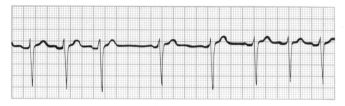

Note: Marked variation in R–R interval.
          Constant PR interval.
          Constant shape of P wave and QRS complex.

   Sinus arrhythmia becomes less marked with increasing age, and it is lost in conditions such as diabetic autonomic neuropathy where vagus nerve function is impaired.
   Extrasystoles. Supraventricular extrasystoles, either atrial or junctional, are commonly seen in normal people and are of no significance.

SUPRAVENTRICULAR EXTRASYSTOLES

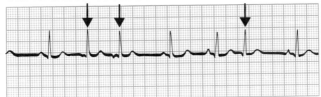

Note: In supraventricular extrasystoles the QRS
complexes and T waves are the same as in the
sinus beats.
Atrial extrasystoles have an abnormal P wave.
Junctional extrasystoles have no P wave.

Ventricular extrasystoles are also commonly seen
in normal ECGs; their significance will be discussed in
Chapter 2.

VENTRICULAR EXTRASYSTOLES

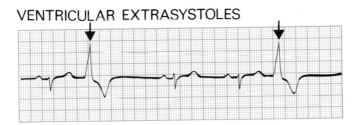

Note: The ventricular extrasystoles are identified by
the absence of a P wave, and the abnormal
QRS complex and T wave.

The P wave

In sinus rhythm the P wave is normally upright in all leads except in VR. When the QRS complex is predominantly downward in VL the P wave may also be inverted.

NORMAL ECG

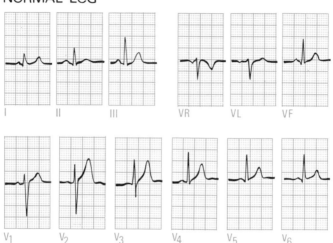

| I | II | III | VR | VL | VF |

| V₁ | V₂ | V₃ | V₄ | V₅ | V₆ |

Note: In both VR and VL the P wave is inverted, and the QRS complex is predominantly downwards.

In patients with dextrocardia the P wave is inverted in lead I although in practice this is more often seen when the limb electrodes have been wrongly attached.

DEXTROCARDIA

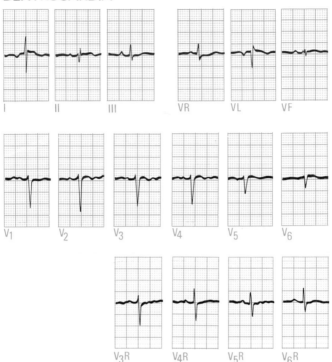

Note: In dextrocardia the P wave is inverted in lead I.
The chest leads V_1—V_6 show right ventricular
complexes.
Electrodes placed on the right side of the chest
in positions corresponding to the normal V
leads on the left side show that the left
ventricle underlies the V_6 position on the right
side of the chest (V_6R).

The PR interval

The PR interval is constant, and the normal range is
0.12–0.22 s (3–5 small squares of ECG paper).

NORMAL ECG

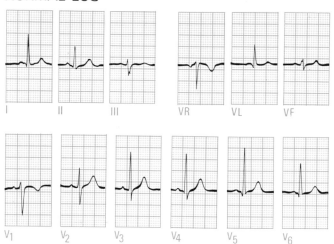

Note: Sinus rhythm; the PR interval is constant in all
leads at 0.16 S.

A PR interval of less than 0.12 s suggests pre-excitation, and a PR interval longer than 0.22 s is due to first degree block: these will be discussed further in Chapter 2.

The QRS complex

The cardiac axis. There is a wide range of normality in the cardiac axis. In most people the QRS complex is tallest in lead II, but in leads I and III the QRS is also predominantly upright (ie the R wave is greater than the S wave).

NORMAL ECG

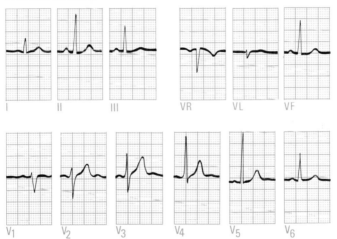

I   II   III   VR   VL   VF

V₁   V₂   V₃   V₄   V₅   V₆

Note: With a normal cardiac axis the QRS complex is predominantly upright in leads I, II and III but is tallest in lead II.

The cardiac axis is still normal when the R wave and
S wave are equal in lead I: this pattern is common in
tall subjects.

NORMAL ECG

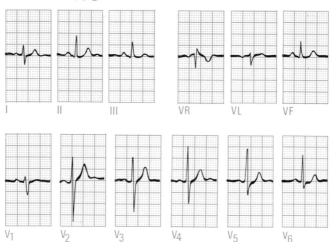

Note: The record shows the limit of normality of the
cardiac axis.

The R and S waves are equal in lead I.

When the S wave exceeds the R wave in lead I right axis deviation is present (see Ch. 4).

It is common for the S wave to exceed the R wave in lead III, and it is acceptable for the S to equal the R in lead II; this pattern is common in fat people, and during pregnancy.

NORMAL ECG

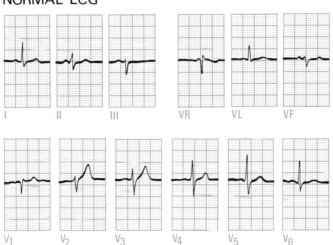

I   II   III   VR   VL   VF

V_1 V_2 V_3 V_4 V_5 V_6

Note: This record shows the limit of normality of the QRS axis.

The S wave exceeds the R wave in lead III.

The S wave equals the R wave in lead II.

When the depth of the S wave exceeds the height of the R wave in lead II, left axis deviation is present (see Chs. 2 and 6).

The size of R and S waves. In lead V_1 there should be a small R wave and a deep S, and the balance between the two should change progressively from V_1 to V_6. In V_6 there should be a tall R wave and no S wave.

NORMAL ECG

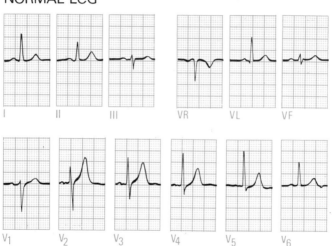

Note: This record shows normal QRS complexes in the V leads. There is progressive change of pattern from V_1 to V_6, with R and S waves equal in V_3.

Very occasionally the ECG of a totally normal subject will show a 'dominant R' (that is, the height of the R exceeds the depth of the S) in V_1.

NORMAL ECG

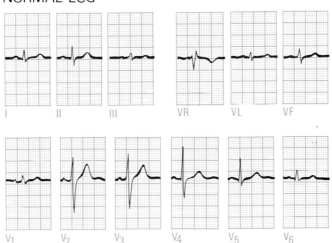

Note: In V_1 the height of the R wave exceeds the depth of the S wave.

However, the presence of a dominant R in V_1 is more likely to be due to either right ventricular hypertrophy or a true posterior infarction (see Chs. 4 and 3).

Although the balance between the height of the R wave and the depth of the S wave is significant for the calculation of cardiac axis and for the identification of right ventricular hypertrophy, the absolute height of the R wave provides little useful information. It is, of course, important that the ECG is properly calibrated with 1 mV = 1 cm of vertical deflection on the ECG. The normal limit is sometimes set at 25 mm for the R wave in V_5 or V_6, or for the S in V_1 or V_2, and the sum of the R in V_5 or V_6 plus the S in V_1 or V_2 is supposed to be less than 35 mm. However, tall R waves in V_5 and V_6 are commonly seen in fit and thin young people and they are perfectly normal.

NORMAL ECG

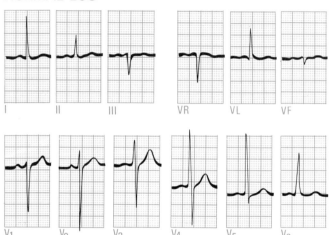

Note: Normal ECG from a young man.
R wave in lead V_5 is 28 mm high, and the S in V_2 is 28 mm deep.

The width of the QRS complex. The QRS complex should be less than 3 mm across (that is, its duration is less than 0.12 S) in all leads. If it is wider than this then either the ventricles have been depolarised from a ventricular rather than a supraventricular focus, (ie, ventricular rhythm is present) or there is an abnormality of conduction within the ventricles. The latter is most commonly due to bundle branch block.

An RSR pattern in V_1, resembling that of right bundle branch block but with a narrow QRS complex, is sometimes called 'partial right bundle branch block' and this is a normal variant.

NORMAL ECG

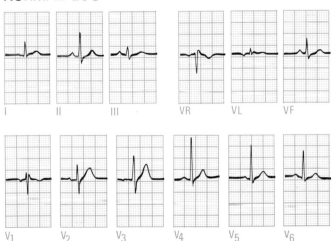

Note: Partial right bundle branch block.
RSR complex in V_1 with QRS duration 0.12 S.

Q waves. The normal depolarisation of the interventricular septum from left to right causes a small 'septal' Q wave in any of leads II, VL and V_5—V_6. Such normal Q waves are less than 2 mm deep and less than 1 mm across.

NORMAL ECG

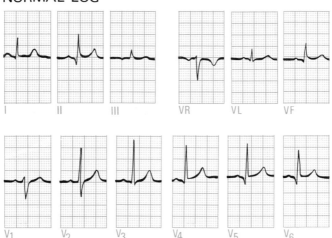

I   II   III   VR   VL   VF

V_1 V_2 V_3 V_4 V_5 V_6

Note: Normal depolarisation of the septum causes small Q waves in leads II, V_5 and V_6.

A small Q wave is also common is lead III; when normal such a Q wave is always narrow, but can occasionally be more than 2 mm deep. These Q waves usually disappear with deep inspiration due to movement of the heart.

NORMAL ECG

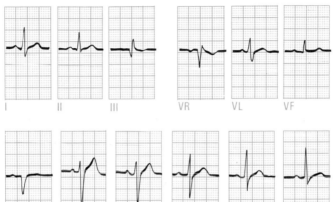

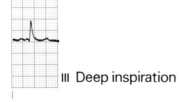

III Deep inspiration

Note: Normal Q waves in lead III.
        No Q wave in lead VF.
        Q wave disappears on inspiration.

When a Q wave is present in lead VF as well as lead III an inferior infarction is likely (see Ch. 3).

The ST segment. The ST segment (the part of the ECG between the S wave and the T wave) should be horizontal and 'isoelectric', which means that it should be at the same level on the paper as the baseline of the record between the end of the T wave and the next P wave.

NORMAL ECG

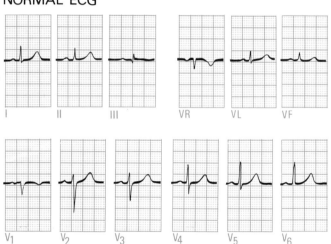

Note: In all leads the ST segment is isoelectric.

An elevation of the ST segment is the hallmark of an acute myocardial infarction, and depression of the ST segment can indicate ischaemia or the effect of digitalis. However, it is perfectly normal for the ST segment to be elevated following an S wave in leads $V_{2, 3}$ and $_4$; this is sometimes called the 'high take-off ST segment'.

NORMAL ECG

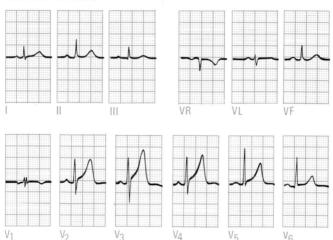

Note: In V_2–V_5 the ST segment is elevated following an S wave.

The T wave. In normal ECGs the T wave is always inverted in VR, but is usually upright in all other leads.

NORMAL ECG

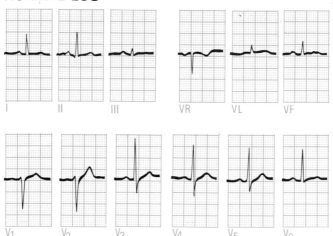

Note: Inverted T wave in VR but the T is upright in all other leads.

The T wave is often inverted in lead III, but becomes more upright on inspiration (see above). The T wave is also often inverted in V₁.

NORMAL ECG

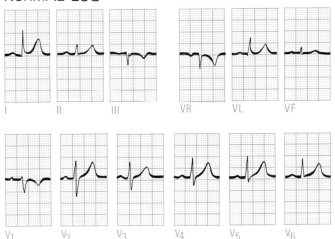

Note: The T wave is inverted in leads III, VR and V₁.

T inversion in V_2 as well as V_1 occurs in right ventricular hypertrophy, but it can be a normal variant and particularly so in black people.

NORMAL ECG (BLACK WOMAN)

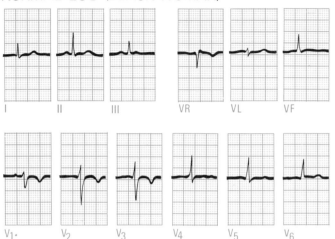

Note: ECG from a black person.
The T wave is inverted in V_1, V_2 and also V_3.

Generalised flattening of the T waves with a normal
QT interval is best described as 'non-specific'.

NORMAL ECG

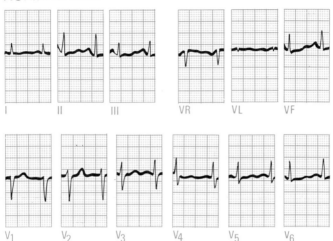

I   II   III   VR   VL   VF

V₁   V₂   V₃   V₄   V₅   V₆

Note: The T waves show non-specific flattening in
          several leads.

Peaked T waves are characteristic of hyperkalaemia, but they are also common in healthy people.

NORMAL ECG

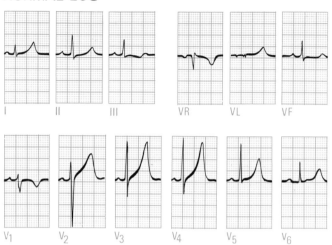

Note: Peaked T waves in V_2–V_4.

An extra hump on the end of the T wave, a 'U' wave, is characteristic of hypokalaemia, but U waves are commonly seen in the anterior chest leads of normal ECGs.

NORMAL ECG

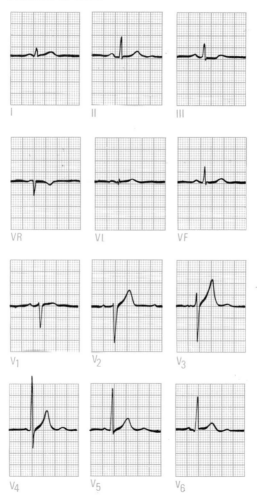

Note: Prominent U waves in V_3, V_4 and V_5.

The ECG in children

The normal heart rate in the first year of life is 140-160 per minute, and it falls slowly to about 80 per minute by puberty. Sinus arrhythmia is usually quite marked in children.

At birth the muscle of the right ventricle is as thick as that in the left ventricle, and the normal ECG of a child in the first year of life has a pattern that would indicate right ventricular hypertrophy in an adult.

NORMAL ECG: AT BIRTH

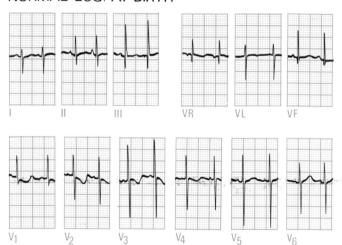

I   II   III   VR   VL   VF

V_1 V_2 V_3 V_4 V_5 V_6

Note: Sinus rhythm, 160 per minute.
Right axis deviation.
Dominant R in V_1.
Deep S wave in V_5.
Inverted T V_1–V_4.

These features gradually disappear.

NORMAL ECG: AGE 1 YEAR

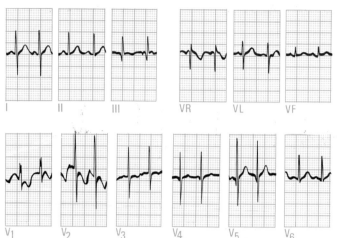

Note: Sinus rhythm, 150 per minute.
Right axis deviation.
Dominant R in V_1.
Inverted T V_1–V_3.

NORMAL ECG: AGE 2 YEARS

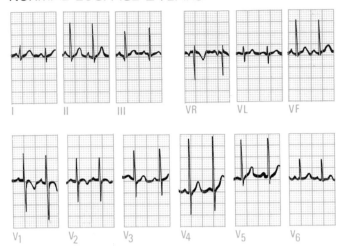

Note: Normal axis.
         S wave exceeds R wave in V_1.
         Inverted T V_1–V_2.

There is obviously some variation in the age at which the apparent right ventricular hypertrophy disappears, but all the features other than the inverted T waves in V_1–V_2 should have disappeared by age 2. The T wave 'abnormalities' may persist to age 10.

NORMAL ECG: AGE 5 YEARS

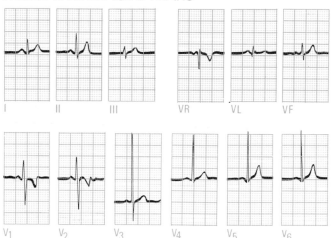

Note: Normal axis.
Normal QRS in the V leads.
T inverted V_1–V_2.

· By the age of 10 the ECG should have taken on the adult pattern.

NORMAL ECG: AGE 10 YEARS

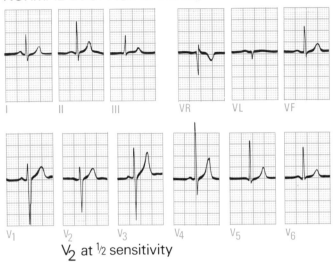

V_2 at ½ sensitivity

Note: The record is indistinguishable from that of a normal adult.

In general, if the infant pattern persists beyond age 2 then right ventricular hypertrophy is indeed present. If the adult pattern is present in the first year of life then left ventricular hypertrophy is present.

Specific ECG abnormalities in healthy people

The ECG findings we have discussed so far can all be considered to be within the normal variation of the

ECG. Certain findings are undoubtedly abnormal so far as the ECG is concerned, yet do occur in apparently healthy people. The frequency with which various abnormalities are detected depends on the population studied: most abnormalities are found least often in healthy young people recruited to the armed services, but become progressively more common in populations of increasing age.

The frequency of right and left bundle branch block has been found respectively to be 0.3% and 0.1% in populations of young recruits, but in older working populations these abnormalities have been described in 2% and 0.7% of apparently healthy people.

Table 1.1 shows the frequency with which the more common ECG abnormalities were encountered in a large survey of civil servants.

Table 1.1   Prevalence of the more common ECG abnormalities in 18 000 civil servants (rates per 1000). (Adapted from Rose et al 1978 British Heart Journal 40: 636–643)

	Age		
	40–49	50–59	60–64
Frequent ventricular extrasystoles	8	14	26
Atrial fibrillation	2	4	11
Left axis deviation	23	32	49
First degree block	18	26	33
LBBB	9	16	31
Abnormal T wave inversion	9	54	76
WPW syndrome	0.3	0.2	0

All the abnormalities, other than the Wolff-Parkinson-White syndrome which is congenital (Ch. 2) were found more frequently with increasing age, suggesting that the various abnormalities are all indicators of heart disease. The survey was of a working population, but some individuals had symptoms of heart disease and of course this was more common in the older age group. This sort of survey shows how difficult it is to know the precise range of 'normality' in the ECG.

What to do

It is essential to recognise the range of normality of the ECG to avoid making a diagnosis of heart disease in a healthy individual. When a specific ECG abnormality is encountered it is important that the subject is not unnecessarily alarmed. In general, an individual's prognosis is not much affected by the ECG abnormality provided he is asymptomatic and his heart is clinically normal. For example, the presence of left bundle branch block in the ECG of an apparently healthy person increases the risk of premature death by a factor of about 1.5 (although of course the absolute risk remains very low) while right bundle branch block has little or no effect on prognosis. However, the combination of symptoms or signs suggesting cardiovascular disease and an abnormal ECG can indicate a higher than average risk.

If an unexpected ECG abnormality is detected it is prudent first to check that the ECG does indeed belong to that patient, and then to take a further history and to check the physical examination; if these are both normal a chest X-ray may be helpful to confirm that the heart is not enlarged and that there are no abnormalities in the pulmonary vasculature, but further investigations are unlikely to reveal any condition that requires treatment.

Although abnormalities in the ECG of apparently healthy people may identify groups of subjects with a somewhat increased risk of developing cardiovascular disease, and thus may be useful in epidemiological studies, the excess of risk is very small in any individual. The ECG is thus not a particularly helpful test in healthy people.

Chapter 2
The ECG in patients with palpitations and syncope

The ECG is of paramount importance for the diagnosis of arrhythmias: no other investigation can substitute for it. Many arrhythmias are not noticed by the patient, and for example they are common in patients who are monitored in a Coronary Care Unit (CCU) following an acute myocardial infarction. However, arrhythmias do sometimes cause symptoms, and frequently these are transient so that the patient is completely well at the time he consults a doctor. Under such circumstances obtaining an ECG during a symptomatic episode is the only certain way of making a diagnosis, but as always the history and physical examination are extremely important.

The clinical history

A cardiac arrhythmia can cause several different symptoms. The patient may become aware of an abnormal heartbeat — the symptom of 'palpitations'. The arrhythmia may interfere with cardiac function and cause dizziness or collapse (syncope) due to hypotension and poor cerebral blood flow, and can also cause breathlessness due to heart failure. Poor coronary blood flow may cause angina.

The main purpose of the history and physical examination is to help decide whether a patient's symptoms could be the result of an arrhythmia, and whether the patient has a cardiac or other disease that might cause an arrhythmia.

Sinus rhythm

People are not normally aware of their heartbeat, but everyone notices the rapid, regular, and forceful beat of sinus tachycardia due to exercise, excitement, or fright. Usually the relationship of such 'palpitations' to a precipitating cause will be obvious, and the individual will not feel the need to seek medical advice. However, anxious subjects may go to their doctor complaining of palpitations which a careful history will show to be due to an enhanced awareness of, and alarm about, a normal heartbeat. Apart from the circumstances in which such 'attacks' occur, the patient will describe a progressive acceleration of heartrate rather than a sudden onset of palpitations. Anxiety-induced sinus tachycardia does not usually compromise cardiac function, though patients with ischaemic heart disease may develop angina. A patient with anxiety-induced sinus tachycardia may complain of breathlessness and dizziness due to hyperventilation, but this can be identified from the typical tingling sensation that this causes around the mouth and in the fingers.

Sinus tachycardia is the appropriate response of the circulation to anaemia, loss of circulating volume, and thyrotoxicosis, and these possible diagnoses must be kept in mind while the history is being taken and the patient examined.

Extrasystoles

Palpitations due to extrasystoles are very common. The patient's description usually makes the diagnosis easy: the heart 'skips a beat', 'jumps into the throat' or 'seems to stop'. Extrasystoles are usually single but may be repeated frequently, and patients tend to notice them particularly when lying in bed at night. Extrasystoles do not cause the symptoms associated with poor cardiac function. Physical examination may reveal an irregularity of the heartbeat, and the only rhythm likely to be confused with extrasystoles is atrial fibrillation. It is not possible to distinguish supraventricular from ventricular extrasystoles either from the history or from the examination.

Paroxysmal tachycardia

An episode of paroxysmal tachycardia typically causes the sudden onset of palpitations. The patient will usually be able to recognise whether the heartbeat is regular or not, and with instruction may be able to count the heart rate. This is valuable information, for a rate less than 140 per minute is usually due to sinus tachycardia. Any unprovoked episode of palpitations associated with chest pain, breathlessness, or dizziness must be considered to be due to an arrhythmia until proved otherwise. If the attack ends abruptly it is almost certainly due to an arrhythmia, though frequently patients will describe episodes of a paroxysmal tachycardia as 'dying away'.

Dizziness and syncope

The most common cause of syncope is simple fainting. This is best recognised from the situations in which attacks occur; the patient is always standing at the time, often in a hot and crowded room or in a situation of emotional stress. A description of the attack from a witness is always helpful: in a faint the patient is pale, the pulse may be difficult to find but if accurately described the heart rate is slow, the rhythm being sinus bradycardia due to vagal overactivity. Recovery occurs within seconds of lying flat.

Syncope can also result from postural hypotension and this is particularly important in old people, in patients taking hypotensive drugs, and in those with abnormalities of autonomic control of the circulation due to diabetes, Parkinsonism, or to idiopathic degeneration of the autonomic nervous system (the Shy-Drager syndrome).

Dizzy attacks or syncope can occur in patients with cardiovascular disease without any abnormality of cardiac rhythm if there is physical obstruction to blood flow. Important causes of such symptoms are aortic stenosis and hypertrophic cardiomyopathy (when dizziness is usually associated with physical activity), intracardiac tumours such as atrial myxomas, and pulmonary embolism. In a young woman, exercise-induced syncope may be caused by severe pulmonary hypertension, sometimes the result of repeated small pulmonary emboli that themselves have caused few symptoms.

The main difficulty, however, is to differentiate syncopal attacks due to arrhythmias from various sorts of epilepsy due to neurological disease, for any syncopal attack due to cerebral hypoxia can cause a grand mal fit. The classical syncopal attack due to an arrhythmia is the 'Stokes Adams' attack associated with complete heart block: here a critical reduction in ventricular rate reduces cardiac output and cerebral flow to the point when sudden loss of consciousness occurs. The patient appears very pale, but flushes red on recovery. Between attacks he may be well, but may describe symptoms of heart failure due to a slow rate. Epileptic attacks due to neurological disease are easy to recognise if there are any features localising to a particular region of the brain, or if there are any associated neurological symptoms between attacks. Frequently, however, this is not the case and differentiation between cardiovascular and neurological disease depends on evidence from examination, or from investigation, of disease in one or other system.

Physical examination

The aim of the physical examination is to find out whether the patient has an arrhythmia, and whether he has any signs of cardiovascular disease that might cause an arrhythmia. An anxious patient complaining of palpitations due to sinus tachycardia will often have a relatively high heart rate (up to 120 or 130 per minute), the skin will be cold and sweaty and the systolic blood pressure will be high. The main differential diagnosis is thyrotoxicosis, which will usually be associated with a goitre and the characteristic warm skin, lid lag, and proptosis. Intermittent attacks of sinus tachycardia occur with phaeocromocytomas, and this diagnosis must be considered when the blood pressure is elevated.

Usually patients with a paroxysmal arrhythmia will be seen when in sinus rhythm, although by chance an arrhythmia may be present at the time of examination. The presence of an abnormality of heart rate or rhythm may give a clue to the nature of paroxysmal attacks, and for example patients with Stokes Adams attacks may be found to be in complete heart block, which can be recognised clinically from the slow and regular heart rate and from the presence of 'cannon' waves in the jugular venous pulse. In young people a slow heart rate may be due to sino atrial disease (the 'sick sinus syndrome') and this can be associated with a paroxysmal tachycardia.

When the patient is in sinus rhythm with a normal heart rate it is necessary to look for some signs of cardiac or (in the case of syncopal attacks) neurological disease. In particular the blood pressure should be measured with the patient both lying and standing, the position of the apex beat should be identified and the presence of right or left ventricular hypertrophy noted. On auscultation it is the presence of aortic and mitral stenosis that are most likely to indicate the cause of syncope or palpitations. Evidence of heart disease of any type makes an arrhythmia a possible cause of palpitations and syncope, but of course arrhythmias commonly cause problems in people whose hearts appear normal between attacks.

The ECG in patients with palpitations and syncope

It is only possible to make a confident diagnosis that an arrhythmia is the cause of palpitations or syncope if an ECG recording of the arrhythmia can be obtained, and if it can be shown that the occurrence of the arrhythmia coincides with the patient's symptoms. If the patient is asymptomatic at the time of examination it may be worth arranging for him to have an ECG recorded immediately any time he has an attack of palpitations, or it may be worth recording the ECG continuously for 24 hours on a tape recorder (the 'Holter' technique) in the hope that an episode of the arrhythmia will be detected. This is relatively time consuming for technicians and is therefore expensive, and it is only worthwhile if there are reasonable clinical grounds for suspecting an arrhythmia, and if the episodes occur sufficiently frequently for there to be a reasonable chance of recording an arrhythmia.

The ECG when the patient is asymptomatic

Syncope due to cardiac causes other than arrhythmias

Although the main use of the ECG is to diagnose arrhythmias, occasionally ECG abnormalities will be seen indictating that syncopal attacks may be due to cardiovascular disease other than an arrhythmia.

The presence of marked left ventricular hypertrophy will suggest the possibility that syncope is due to aortic stenosis.

LV HYPERTROPHY DUE TO AORTIC STENOSIS

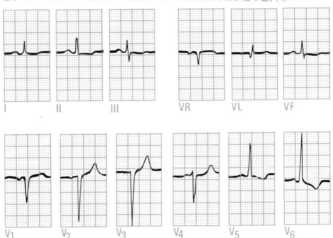

Note: Tall R in V_6, deep S in V_2–V_3.
Inverted T in lead II and V_5—V_6.

ECG evidence of severe right ventricular hypertrophy will raise the possibility of thromboembolic pulmonary hypertension.

RV HYPERTROPHY DUE TO MULTIPLE PULMONARY EMBOLI

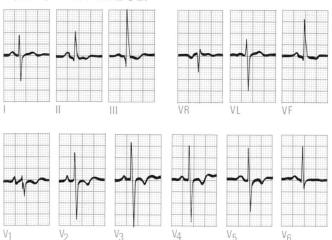

Note: Sinus rhythm.
Peaked P waves
Right axis deviation
Inverted T in V_1–V_5
The only 'missing' feature of right ventricular hypertrophy is a dominant R in V_1 (see Ch. 4).

In addition, however, the ECG may suggest that an arrhythmia is likely even when the patient is asymptomatic and physical examination is normal.

Patients with possible tachycardia

Mitral stenosis. Mitral stenosis is an important cause
of atrial fibrillation, so ECG evidence of mitral
stenosis may indicate that this arrhythmia is the
cause of intermittent irregular and fast palpitations.

MITRAL STENOSIS

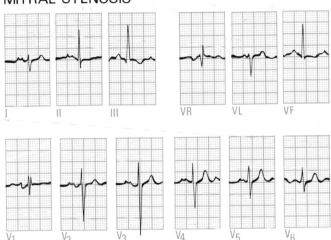

Note: Sinus rhythm
Broad and notched P waves suggest left atrial
hypertrophy.
Right axis deviation and S wave in V_6 suggests
right ventricular hypertrophy.
The partial RBBB is not significant.

Pre-excitation syndromes. In the pre-excitation syndromes there are abnormal pathways connecting the atria and ventricles which form an anatomical basis for re-entry tachycardia (see Ch. 6).

In the *Wolff-Parkinson-White syndrome* an accessory pathway can be identified microscopically: this is usually between the left atrium and left ventricle, but sometimes there is an abnormal connection between the right atrium and ventricle. In either case the normal atrioventricular nodal delay is bypassed so the PR interval is short and ventricular activation is initially abnormal. However excitation spreading through the AV node and bundle of His causes normal late ventricular excitation. A short PR interval is thus followed by a slurred upstroke of the QRS, and this slurring is called a delta wave.

With a left sided accessory pathway the ECG shows a dominant R wave in V_1, and superficially resembles right ventricular hypertrophy (Type A pattern).

WOLFF-PARKINSON-WHITE SYNDROME

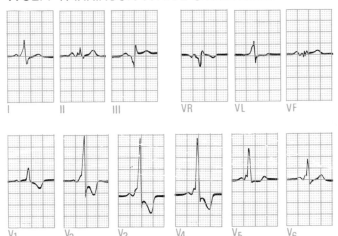

Note: Short PR interval
Slurred upstroke of R wave (delta wave)
Dominant R in V_1
Inverted T V_1–V_4.

When the accessory pathway is on the right side of the heart there is no dominant R in V_1, and this is called 'Type B'.

WOLFF-PARKINSON-WHITE SYNDROME

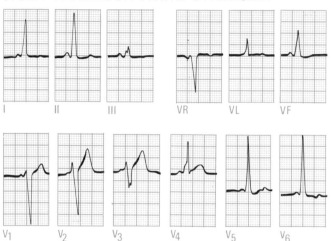

I   II   III   VR   VL   VF

V_1 V_2 V_3 V_4 V_5 V_6

Note: Short PR interval
The delta wave is most obvious in V_4.

Where there is a bypass causing rapid conduction through the AV node itself there is also a short PR interval, but the QRS complex is entirely normal; this is the Lown-Ganong-Levine syndrome.

LOWN-GANONG-LEVINE SYNDROME

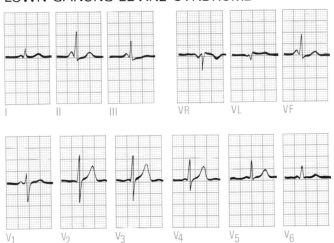

I   II   III   VR   VL   VF

V₁   V₂   V₃   V₄   V₅   V₆

Note: Short PR interval
Narrow and normal QRS complexes

Pre-excitation syndromes are found in approximately 1 of every 3000 healthy young people, and probably only half ever have an episode of tachycardia; many of these only have very occasional attacks. During an episode of re-entry tachycardia the QRS complex is usually narrow and the pattern resembles a junctional tachycardia; the presence of a pre-excitation syndrome may not be suspected.

Broad complex tachycardias also occur in patients with the WPW syndrome. Although the ECG may resemble ventricular tachycardia, in most cases the underlying rhythm is probably atrial fibrillation with anomalous atrioventricular conduction. This is a serious arrhythmia, for ventricular fibrillation may occur.

TACHYCARDIAS IN WPW SYNDROME

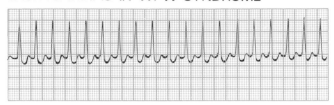

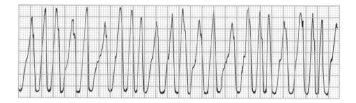

Note: Upper trace shows a narrow complex, and lower trace shows a wide complex, tachycardia. The underlying diagnosis of WPW syndrome is not apparent in either case.

The long QT syndrome. Delayed repolarisation occasionally occurs for no apparent reason; the ECG shows a prolonged QT interval but of itself this does not impair cardiac function and does not cause symptoms. The prolonged QT interval, is however, sometimes associated with paroxysmal ventricular tachycardia.

LONG QT SYNDROME

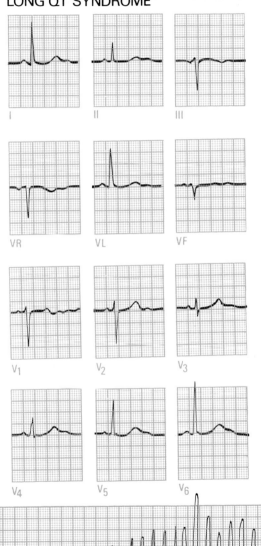

Note: Sinus rhythm with a normal PR interval and a normal cardiac axis.
The T wave is followed by a U wave, and the Q–U interval is 0.72 sec.
The patient had frequent episodes of ventricular tachycardia (bottom strip).

Patients with possible bradycardias

When the patient is asymptomatic an intermittent bradycardia can be suspected if the ECG shows any evidence of a conduction defect. Nevertheless, it must be remembered that conduction defects are quite common in the healthy population, and their presence may be coincidental. (Ch. 1).

Intermittent complete heart block is, however, more likely to occur when there is evidence of abnormal conduction in two of the three main divisions of the bundle of His (the right bundle and the anterior and posterior divisions of the left bundle branch). 'Bifascicular block' is indicated by the combination of right bundle branch block and marked left axis deviation.

BIFASCICULAR BLOCK

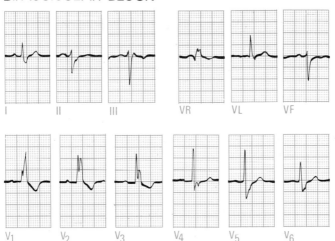

I   II   III   VR   VL   VF

V₁   V₂   V₃   V₄   V₅   V₆

Note: Sinus rhythm
         Left axis deviation
         QRS complex shows RSR pattern in V₁
         indicating right bundle branch block (RBBB).

The combination of bundle branch block and first degree block also suggests conduction may intermittently fail in the remaining bundle branch.

1st DEGREE BLOCK AND BUNDLE BRANCH BLOCK

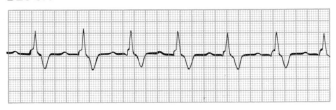

Note: PR interval 0.28 s indicating first degree block. Broad QRS and inverted T wave indicates bundle branch block, but it is not possible to tell from a single lead which branch is affected.

The ECG when the patient has symptoms

Several arrhythmias are of considerable physiological interest but do not cause symptoms: these will be discussed in Chapter 6. If an ECG can be recorded at the time when the patient has palpitations, dizziness, or syncope then there can be little doubt about the relation between the symptoms and the cardiac rhythm.

Sinus rhythm

When sinus tachycardia results from anxiety, heart rates of up to 150 per minute are not uncommon. The rhythm may be mistaken for an atrial tachycardia but pressure on the carotid sinus will cause transient slowing of the heart rate and the P waves will become more obvious.

Marked sinus bradycardia is characteristic of athletic training, but it is part of the cause of symptoms in fainting (the 'vasovagal' attack) and it may also contribute to hypotension and heart failure in a patient with an inferior myocardial infarction.

Extrasystoles

An ECG is necessary to differentiate between supraventricular and ventricular extrasystoles.

When extrasystoles have a supraventricular origin the QRS complex is narrow, and both it and the T wave have the same configuration as the sinus beat. Atrial extrasystoles have abnormal P waves, and junctional extrasystoles either have a P wave very close to the QRS complex (in front of it or behind it) or no P waves may be visible.

ATRIAL EXTRASYSTOLE

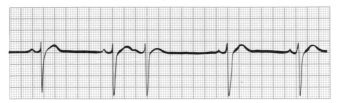

JUNCTIONAL (NODAL) EXTRASYSTOLE

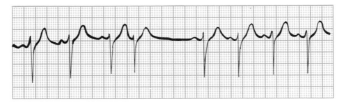

Note: An atrial extrasystole has an abnormally
shaped P wave.
A junctional (AV nodal) extrasystole usually
shows no P wave.

Ventricular extrasystoles are wide and have an abnormal shape, and the T wave is also usually abnormal. No P waves are present.

VENTRICULAR EXTRASYSTOLES

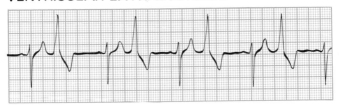

Note: Each sinus beat is followed by a beat with no P wave, a wide QRS and an inverted T wave. This is sometimes called 'bigeminy'.

The corresponding 'escape beats' have the same characteristics but occur late rather than early (see Ch. 6).

When a ventricular extrasystole appears on the upstroke of the T wave of the preceding beat, the 'R on T' phenomenon is said to be present. This can initiate ventricular fibrillation, but usually it does not do so.

R ON T PHENOMENON

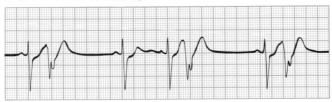

Note: Ventricular extrasystoles occur near the peak of the preceding T wave.

Tachycardias

Supraventricular tachycardias. Properly speaking, sinus, atrial and junctional arrhythmias are all 'supraventricular', but the term 'supraventricular tachycardia' is often inappropriately used interchangeably with junctional tachycardia. All these supraventricular rhythms have QRS complexes of normal shape and width, and the T waves have the same shape as the sinus beat.

In *atrial tachycardia* P waves are present, sometimes hidden in the T wave of the preceding beat.

ATRIAL TACHYCARDIA

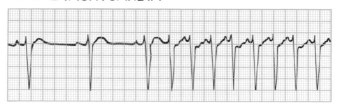

Note: Two sinus beats are followed by a sudden change of heart rate. In the tachycardia P waves can be seen as humps on the T waves of the preceding beats.

When the atrial rate exceeds about 180 per minute physiological block will occur in the atrioventricular node so that the ventricular rate becomes half that of the atrium. The main importance of atrial tachycardia with 2:1 block is that it is characteristic of digitalis toxicity.

In *atrial flutter* the atrial rate is about 300 per minute, and the P waves form a continuous 'saw-tooth' line. Because the AV node fails to conduct all the P waves the relationship between P waves and QRS complexes is usually 2:1, 3:1, or 4:1.

ATRIAL FLUTTER
2:1 block

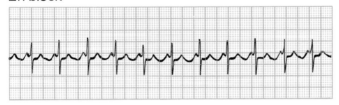

4:1 block

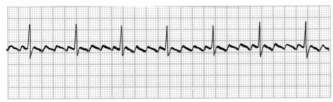

Note: In atrial flutter with 2:1 block a P wave may be confused with a T wave. With 4:1 block the flutter waves are obvious.

With 2:1 conduction the 'saw-tooth' may not be obvious in all leads, and as always it is best to examine a 12 lead cardiogram and diagnose the rhythm from the lead in which the P waves are most obvious.

ATRIAL FLUTTER

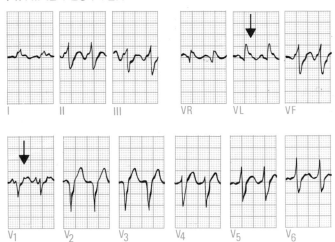

Note: In this record the P waves are most obvious in leads VL and V_1.

If the ventricular rate is rapid, carotid sinus pressure will usually increase the block at the AV node and make the 'saw-tooth' more obvious, (see p.91).

In *junctional tachycardia* no P waves can be seen. Carotid sinus pressure either reverts the heart to sinus rhythm, or has no effect.

JUNCTIONAL TACHYCARDIA

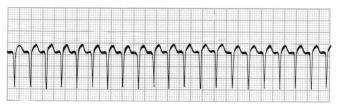

Note: Regular narrow QRS complexes at 180 per minute.
No P waves visible.

In *atrial fibrillation* disorganised atrial activity causes the P waves to disappear, and the ECG baseline becomes totally irregular. At times atrial activity may become sufficiently synchronised for a 'flutter-like' pattern to appear, but this rapidly breaks up. The QRS complexes are totally irregular.

ATRIAL FIBRILLATION

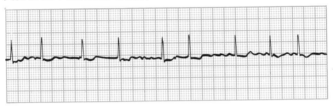

Note: Variable atrial activity with 'flutter' waves at times.
Irregular narrow QRS complexes.

The QRS complex may become regular seen with digitalis toxicity. It is important to remember that totally regular and slow, QRS complexes may indicate complete heart block and this can occur in the presence of atrial fibrillation.

ATRIAL FIBRILLATION WITH COMPLETE BLOCK

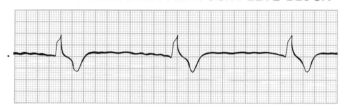

Note: Variable atrial activity
Regular wide QRS complexes at 30 per minute.

Ventricular tachycardia. Ventricular tachycardia causes an ECG with wide and abnormal QRS complexes and abnormal T waves; the heart rate is greater than 120 per minute. Rhythms of ventricular origin with lower rates are due to accelerated idioventricular rhythm (see Ch. 6). Although ventricular tachycardia often causes marked dizziness, chest pain, or breathlessness it can be relatively asymptomatic, and it is not safe to assume that a paroxysmal tachycardia that does not apparently cause haemodynamic impairment cannot be ventricular in origin.

VENTRICULAR TACHYCARDIA

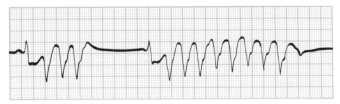

Note: A sinus beat is followed by 3 ventricular beats at 210 per minute.
A second sinus beat is followed by a run of ventricular tachycardia.

The diagnosis of broad complex tachycardias.
Tachycardias in which the QRS complexes are broad
(greater than 0.12 s) are usually ventricular in origin,
but occasionally they may be supraventricular with
the broad QRS being the result of bundle branch
block. The combination of supraventricular
tachycardia and bundle branch block may
occur if conduction down one or other bundle
branch is somewhat impaired: conduction can be
normal at normal heart rates, but block
('rate-dependent bundle branch block') may occur at
high heart rates.

It is only safe to assume that a broad complex
tachycardia has a supraventricular origin when it can
be shown that bundle branch block is present when
the patient is in sinus rhythm, and that the QRS
complex has the same shape during the tachycardia
that it has in sinus rhythm.

SUPRAVENTRICULAR TACHYCARDIA WITH BUNDLE BRANCH BLOCK

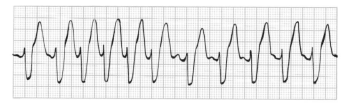

Note: This record shows a single sinus beat with a
broad QRS, followed by 5 beats without P
waves but with the same broad QRS complex.
Sinus rhythm is then restored. This arrhythmia
is junctional tachycardia with bundle branch
block.

When a patient has a sustained broad complex tachycardia the most helpful piece of information may be an ECG recorded on some previous occasion.

SINUS RHYTHM WITH BIFASCICULAR BLOCK

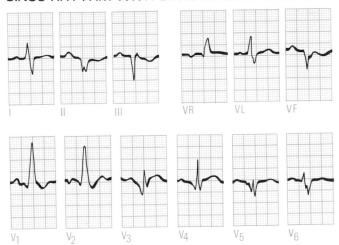

Note: Sinus rhythm with left axis deviation. Broad QRS complexes with an RSR pattern in V_1 and a deep notched S in V_6 indicate RBBB.

SUPRAVENTRICULAR TACHYCARDIA

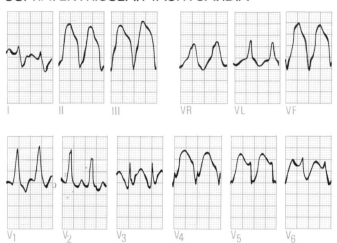

Note: The same patient during an episode of
tachycardia. Unless it were known that the
same ECG appearance was present in sinus
rhythm it would have been assumed that this
is ventricular tachycardia.

The ECG may, however, give other clues. If an early beat can be found with a narrow QRS it can be assumed that a wide complex tachycardia is ventricular in origin, for the narrow early beat demonstrates that the bundle branches will conduct supraventricular beats normally, even at high heart rates.

VENTRICULAR TACHYCARDIA

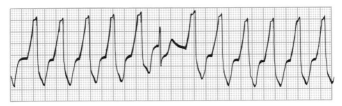

Note: A single early beat with a narrow QRS interrupts a broad complex tachycardia. The single beat must have a supraventricular origin, and by implication the broad complexes must have a ventricular origin.

Occasionally it may be possible to identify P waves at a slower rate than the QRS complexes.

VENTRICULAR TACHYCARDIA

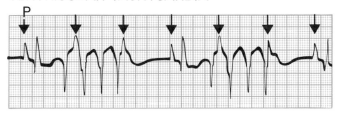

Note: A single sinus beat is followed by a broad complex tachycardia. During the tachycardia P waves can still be seen at a normal rate, so the broad complex tachycardia must have a ventricular origin.

A deep S wave in V_6 makes it likely that a broad complex tachycardia is ventricular in origin. A dominant R in V_1 *without* a deep S in V_6 suggests that the rhythm is supraventricular.

Usually P waves cannot be seen in the ordinary ECG during a broad complex tachycardia, but atrial activity can be demonstrated by passing a pacing catheter percutaneously to the right atrium, and recording from the catheter simultaneously with a surface ECG on a 2-channel recorder. In an intracardiac recording the atrial activity is said to cause an 'A' wave and ventricular activity a 'V' wave.

SINUS RHYTHM
Surface ECG

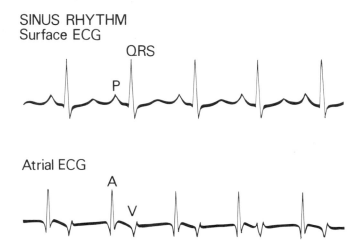

Atrial ECG

Note: Upper trace shows the normal surface ECG. Lower trace is recorded simultaneously from a pacing wire in the right atrium. The 'A' wave (corresponding to the P wave in the surface ECG) appears much larger than the 'V' (which corresponds to the QRS complex).

VENTRICULAR TACHYCARDIA
Lead II

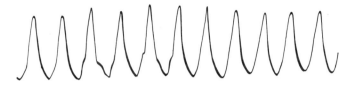

Atrial ECG

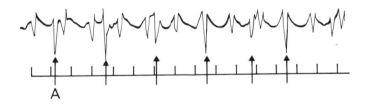

Note: In ventricular tachycardia 'A' waves can be seen in the right atrial trace, at a slower rate and completely dissociated from the 'V' waves.

The presence of dissociated P waves proves that the rhythm has a ventricular origin. However, associated (1:1) P waves can occur in ventricular rhythms if the atria are activated retrogradely up the His Bundle.

Recording an intracardiac ECG is safe and simple, provided the appropriate equipment is available. However, it only becomes necessary when a patient has recurrent attacks of a broad complex tachycardia that are refractory to treatment.

Remember that a broad complex tachycardia is nearly always ventricular in origin. Remember also that a patient may withstand a ventricular tachycardia relatively well for a while, and that it is not safe to assume that a rhythm must have a supraventricular origin because the patient looks well.

VENTRICULAR TACHYCARDIA

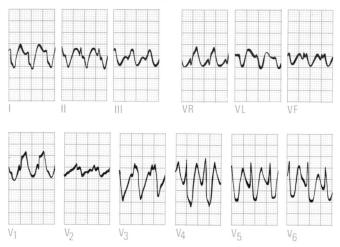

Note: Broad complex tachycardia: although in some leads deflections can be seen that could be P waves they could equally well be part of a broad QRS.

Assume that a broad complex tachycardia is ventricular tachycardia until proved otherwise.

Ventricular flutter and fibrillation. Very rapid ventricular tachycardia is sometimes called 'ventricular flutter'; this rhythm seldom supports an effective cardiac output.

VENTRICULAR "FLUTTER"

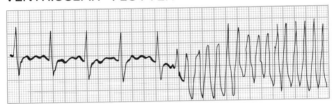

Note: Five sinus beats are followed by ventricular tachycardia at 300 per minute — sometimes called 'ventricular flutter'.

This has much the same effect as, and usually degenerates to, ventricular fibrillation.

VENTRICULAR FIBRILLATION

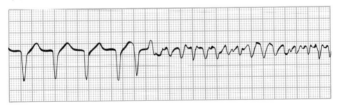

Note: The T wave of the fourth sinus beat is interrupted by a ventricular extrasystole (the 'R on T' phenomenon). This is followed by the chaotic trace of ventricular fibrillation.

Bradycardias

In this chapter we are primarily concerned with arrhythmias that cause symptoms; rhythms that are mainly of physiological interest are discussed in Chapter 6. This separation is, however, to some extent artificial for whether or not an arrhythmia causes symptoms to some extent depends on how frequently it occurs.

The sick sinus syndrome. Supraventricular escape rhythms that occur intermittently are often asymptomatic, and are described in Chapter 6. They characterise the 'sick sinus syndrome', a condition in which abnormal sinus node function may be associated with other abnormalities in the conducting system. Disordered sinus node function can be familial or congenital, can occur in ischaemic, rheumatic, hypertensive or infiltrative cardiac disease, but it is frequently idiopathic. The patient may be asymptomatic, but bradycardias can cause symptoms of heart failure and dizziness, and since atrial and junctional tachycardias often occur the patient may present with palpitations. The combination of sick sinus syndrome and tachycardias is sometimes called the 'bradycardia-tachycardia syndrome'. Rhythms that may be seen in this syndrome include 'sinus pauses' (sinus arrest and sinoatrial block) — see Chapter 6 — and also atrial standstill (the 'silent atrium'). This is a common presentation and the rhythm is maintained by junctional escape beats.

SICK SINUS SYNDROME

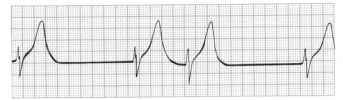

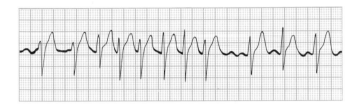

Note: Upper trace shows a 'silent atrium' with
irregular junctional escape beats.
With this rhythm the patient was
asymptomatic but he had episodes of
junctional tachycardia (lower trace) which
caused him to complain of palpitations. In the
lower trace junctional tachycardia is followed
by a period of sinus rhythm.

The prognosis of the sick sinus syndrome is that of the underlying disease, and patients with an idiopathic condition do well.

Atrioventricular block. Atrioventricular block can complicate any cardiac disease. It is common, and usually temporary, in acute myocardial infarction. Chronic heart block, particularly in elderly people, is usually a manifestation of fibrotic degeneration of the conducting system rather than of ischaemic heart disease.

First degree block, and second degree block of the Wenckebach and Mobitz 2 variety, are asymptomatic. While they are indicators of heart disease and are of physiological interest they are not of themselves clinically important (see Ch. 6). Second degree AV block with 2:1 atrioventricular conduction may cause symptoms if the ventricular rate is low enough.

Complete, or third degree, atrioventricular block can be asymptomatic, or may cause heart failure. If the ventricular rate slows below a critical level the patient may lose consciousness in a Stokes Adams attack.

COMPLETE BLOCK AND STOKES-ADAMS ATTACK

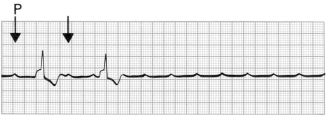

Note: After 2 complexes ventricular activity ceases, leaving only P waves. After a few seconds the patient lost consciousness in a Stokes Adams attack.

The ECG in patients with pacemakers

Patients with bradycardias may be treated by the insertion of a temporary or permanent pacemaker. Occasionally the electrode that connects the pulse generator ('the battery') to the heart is sewn onto the epicardium, but usually a 'wire' is inserted via a vein in the neck, through the right atrium and tricuspid valve, so that the electrode at its tip comes into contact with the endocardium of the right ventricle. For some special purposes two electrodes may be inserted to allow stimulation of both the right atrium and the right ventricle.

Right ventricular stimulation maintains cardiac function because excitation spreads through the Purkinje system to the left ventricle. The rhythm is thus 'ventricular' in origin, and the ECG shows a broad and abnormal QRS complex with an abnormal T wave. The electrical discharge of the pacemaker is recorded as a 'pacing spike' immediately before the QRS complex.

PACED RHYTHM

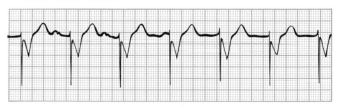

Note: The pacemaker stimulus causes a well defined brief spike (often not as well seen as in this record) and this is followed immediately by a broad 'ventricular' QRS complex.

Early pacemakers were 'fixed rate' which meant that they produced pacing impulses at a constant frequency, independent of any spontaneous cardiac activities. The patient's own rhythm and that of the pacemaker could therefore compete.

FIXED RATE PACING
Pacemaker on

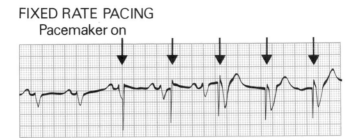

Note: After two sinus beats the pacemaker is switched on. The first pacing spike corresponds with a QRS complex and the second with the T wave of a sinus beat: neither impulse stimulates the ventricle. A third pacing spike interrupts the T wave of a sinus beat but the ventricles are stimulated and two further paced beats follow. The arrival of a pacemaker impulse on a T wave could precipitate ventricular fibrillation but did not do so in this case.

All pacemakers are now of the 'demand' type, which means that they sense any spontaneous ventricular depolarisation and this inhibits the pacemaker. Thus if the pacemaker is set at a demand rate of 60 per minute it will delay for 1 second after any spontaneous heartbeat; this means that the heart rate will never fall below 60 per minute, but the rate may exceed this if spontaneous depolarisation occurs more frequently.

"DEMAND" PACING

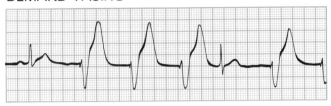

Note: After a sinus beat there is no cardiac activity for 0.92 seconds. The pacemaker is then activated at its preset rate of 70 per minute, but it is designed not to initiate pacing until a pause slightly longer than there is between paced beats. After 4 paced beats a single sinus beat inhibits the pacemaker, but after a further pause of 0.92 seconds the pacemaker is again activated.

Some modern pacemakers are 'programmable', which means that their rate and some other characteristics of the impulse they produce can be changed by an external 'programmer' after the pacemaker has been inserted. Progressively more sophisticated pacemakers are being introduced, and one variant allows 'sequential' pacing of the right atrium and ventricle so that the atrial contribution to cardiac output is maintained.

What to do

What to do when an arrhythmia is suspected

24 hour (ambulatory) ECG monitoring. The only way to be certain that a patient's symptoms are due to an arrhythmia is to record an ECG at the time of the attack. When symptoms are intermittent and infrequent this can be extremely difficult.

If the patient has symptoms at some time during most days it is certainly worth recording the ECG continuously on a portable tape recorder while the patient carries on with his or her normal activity. This is called 'ambulatory' or 'Holter' monitoring, after the inventor of the initial recorder. Making and analysing these records is relatively expensive in technician time, and it is seldom helpful if the patient has symptoms less than once in every two or three weeks.

If a patient records the presence of symptoms at a time when the ECG shows an arrhythmia, it is safe to assume that the symptoms and the arrhythmia are related. The following records were all obtained from patients who complained of palpitations or syncope, but who were in sinus rhythm at the time when they were examined and their resting ECGs were normal.

24HR RECORD. SUPRAVENTRICULAR EXTRASYSTOLES

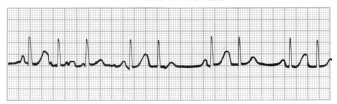

Note: Frequent supraventricular extrasystoles recorded at the time when the patient had palpitations.

Occasionally a 24 hour ECG recording may show multiple abnormalities and the rhythm associated with a major attack of symptoms may be recorded.

24HR RECORD: STOKES-ADAMS ATTACK

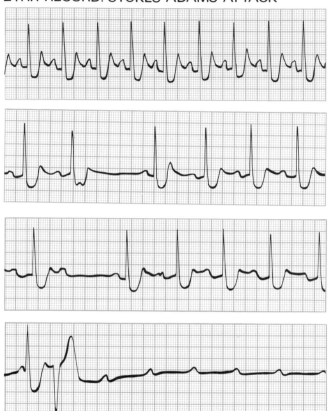

Note: Top strip shows sinus rhythm with normal AV conduction.

Second strip shows sino-atrial block and the third strip shows second degree block — both these were asymptomatic.

Bottom strip shows a ventricular extrasystole followed by complete heart block with ventricular standstill. The patient lost consciousness due to this 'Stokes-Adams' attack.

If the patient has no symptoms during the time the record is being made, and the ECG shows sinus rhythm throughout, the investigation is unhelpful and a decision whether to repeat it depends on clinical judgement. When the patient's story is highly suggestive of an arrhythmia it may be justifiable to make repeated 24 hour records.

THREE 24 HR RECORDS FROM ONE PATIENT

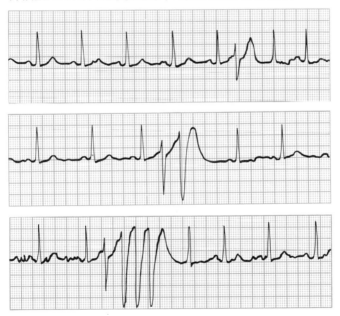

Note: Samples from three separate 24 hour records made at weekly intervals.
Top strip shows sinus rhythm.
Second record shows a couplet of ventricular extrasystoles (no symptoms noted).

Third record shows a short run of ventricular tachycardia which corresponded to the patient's complaint of palpitations.

When the 24 hour ECG shows some arrhythmias which are not accompanied by symptoms, it is very difficult to be certain of their significance. Table 2.1 shows the arrhythmias that were detected during two 24 hour periods in a group of 86 volunteers who were apparently completely free of heart disease. This study shows that supposedly dangerous arrhythmias such as ventricular tachycardia can occur and pass unnoticed in apparently healthy people.

Table 2.1   Arrhythmias observed during 48 hours of ambulatory recording in 86 healthy subjects aged 16-65. (From Clarke et al 1976 Lancet 2: 508-510)

Ventricular extrasystoles		63
Multifocal	13	
Bigeminy	13	
R on T	3	
Ventricular tachycardia		2
Supraventricular tachycardia		4
Junctional escape		8
Second degree block		2

Ventricular extrasystoles are so common that they can clearly be ignored, although epidemiological evidence suggests that in large groups of patients they can be crude 'markers' of heart disease. A few couplets of extrasystoles on a 24 hour record can also be accepted as within the normal range.

24HR RECORD

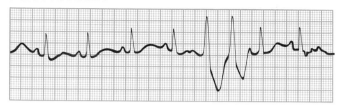

Note: Sinus rhythm with a 'couplet' of ventricular
extrasystoles — no associated symptoms.

Frequent couplets, however, probably do indicate
heart disease. If the patient complains of palpitations
but has no such symptoms even though the record
shows frequent couplets, the occurrence of
ventricular tachycardia must be suspected and either
the record must be repeated or prophylactic
treatment given.

24HR RECORD

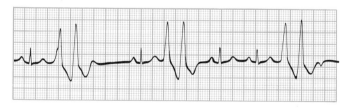

Note: Sinus rhythm with frequent couplets of
ventricular extrasystoles.

Similarly, the intermittent appearance of asymptomatic second degree block must raise the possibility that symptoms may be due to intermittent complete block.

When ventricular extrasystoles occur in runs of three or more the term 'salvoes' is sometimes used, but three or more ventricular extrasystoles together are usually considered to constitute ventricular tachycardia.

24 HR RECORD

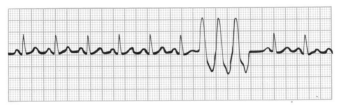

Note: Sinus rhythm with a short run of ventricular tachycardia.

Although even repeated short runs of ventricular tachycardia may not cause symptoms and may be seen in healthy people, they cannot be regarded as insignificant in patients with palpitations or syncope.

24 HR RECORD

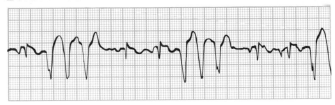

Note: Every two sinus beats are followed by a short run of ventricular tachycardia.

This progression from the asymptomatic and insignificant occasional couplet to the frequent short runs of ventricular tachycardia is clearly gradual, and there is no certain point at which an arrhythmia that does not correspond with symptoms can be described as definitely significant. In any individual patient it can thus be very difficult to know when to begin treatment.

Patients who die suddenly while 24 hour ECG records are being made are usually found to have ventricular fibrillation.

SUDDEN DEATH

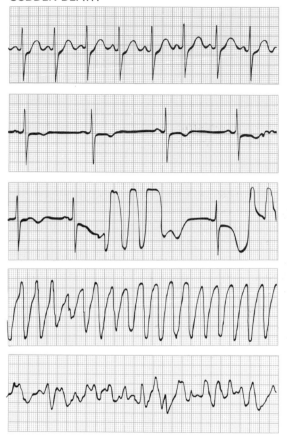

Note: First strip shows sinus rhythm. Sinus
bradycardia develops, with inversion of the T
waves suggesting ischaemia. Short runs of
ventricular tachycardia lead to ventricular
'flutter', and then to ventricular fibrillation.

Precipitation of arrhythmias. Arrhythmias are sometimes precipitated by exercise, and if the patient's history suggests that this is so treadmill testing may be helpful. Attempts to provoke an arrhythmia by exercise, should, however, only be made when full resuscitation facilities are available.

REST

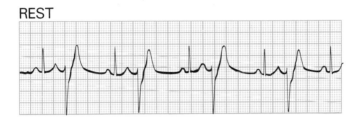

EXERCISE

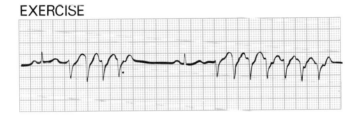

Note: At rest the ECG shows frequent ventricular extrasystoles.
After exercise ventricular tachycardia occurs.

If the patient complains of syncopal attacks, particularly on movement of the head, it is worth pressing the carotid sinus in the neck to see whether the patient has carotid sinus hypersensitivity. Complete sino-atrial node inhibition may be induced, sometimes with unpleasant escape arrhythmias.

CAROTID SINUS HYPERSENSITIVITY

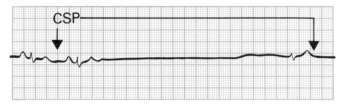

Note: Carotid sinus pressure causes cessation of all cardiac activity due to excess of vagal function.

What to do when an arrhythmia is recorded

The first problem is to decide whether the arrhythmia has a cause that can or should be treated. The most common cause of arrhythmias is acute myocardial infarction, when any arrhythmia may arise; the arrhythmias become progressively less common after the first 24 hours. In some other diseases arrhythmias are characteristic: for example, atrial fibrillation is part of the natural history of chronic rheumatic heart disease and it is also common in alcoholic cardiomyopathy. In old people thyrotoxicosis may present with atrial fibrillation and few other symptoms. Several drugs — notably digoxin and the tricyclic antidepressives — cause arrhythmias, and it is important to remember that all the 'class 1' antiarrhythmic agents (quinidine, disopyramide, flecainide) can also at times precipitate ventricular tachycardia.

The second problem is to decide whether the arrhythmia itself needs treatment. In general, arrhythmias that cause symptoms, or cause hypotension or signs of heart failure, must be treated. Those that have no effect can often be left alone, but some arrhythmias are likely to cause problems unless they are treated, and for example a rapid and sustained supraventricular or ventricular tachycardia needs urgent treatment however well the patient appears to be for deterioration is inevitable.

Since arrhythmias are most commonly encountered in patients with acute myocardial infarction their management can be considered from this viewpoint, but in fact the principles are the same whatever the patient's underlying disease. There are many antiarrhythmic drugs, and all arrhythmias can be treated in more than one way. It is best, however, to use a limited number of drugs in a consistent way so as to get experience with them. What follows is a simple and safe therapeutic policy based on a few drugs.

Principles of arrhythmia management

1. Any arrhythmia causing significant symptoms or a haemodynamic disturbance must be treated immediately.
2. All antiarrhythmic drugs should be considered as cardiac depressants, and some can actually induce arrhythmias. The use of multiple agents should be avoided.
3. Electrical treatment (cardioversion for tachycardias, pacing for bradycardias) should be

used in preference to drug therapy when there is marked haemodynamic impairment.

Cardiac arrest

Remember: Airway
            Breathing
            Cardiac massage

Ventricular fibrillation DC shock at 200J, repeated at 200J then 320J if necessary.
If unsuccessful CPR and
      Bicarbonate 100 mmol × 1—2 (i.e. 100-200 ml of 8.4%)
      Lignocaine 100 mg. IV bolus
      Repeat DC shock at 320 J
   Blood gasses should be checked as soon as it is convenient to do so.

DC CONVERSION OF VENTRICULAR FIBRILLATION
DC shock

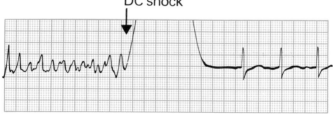

Note: Ventricular fibrillation is abolished by a DC shock and a supraventricular rhythm (probably sinus in origin) immediately takes control of the heart.

It is not necessary to give routine antiarrhythmic
therapy after successful treatment of a first episode of
VF.

Asystole
Precordial thump
Maintain CPR
Isoprenaline 100 micrograms bolus i.v. followed by 1
microgram per minute infusion (2 mg in 500 ml
dextrose — 4 micrograms per ml)
Calcium gluconate 10 ml 10% solution i.v. (= 1 mg).
Bicarbonate 100 ml of 8.4% × 1–2.
If successful, insert temporary pacemaker.

Extrasystoles

Supraventricular — no treatment: if the patient has
symptoms, explanation and reassurance.
Ventricular — usually no treatment, though this may
be considered:
1. When VEs are so frequent that cardiac output is
   impaired.
2. When there is a frequent R on T. phenomenon.
3. Three VEs together should be considered as
   ventricular tachycardia.
4. When the patient complains of an irregular heart
   beat and reassurance and an explanation prove
   ineffective.
Treatment for VEs is as for ventricular tachycardia.

Tachycardias

The first step in the treatment of any tachycardia is
carotid sinus pressure.

In sinus rhythm carotid sinus pressure will cause
transient slowing of the heart rate. This may be useful

to demonstrate the true origin of the rhythm when there is doubt.

CSP AND SINUS RHYTHM

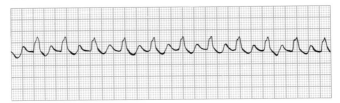

CSP

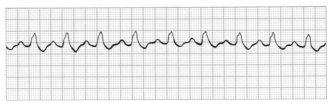

Note: Upper trace shows a broad complex tachycardia and it is not obvious whether the biphasic deflection before the QRS represents a T wave, or a T followed by a P.
Lower record shows the effect of carotid sinus pressure. The rate is slowed and P waves are obvious.

In atrial flutter, atrioventricular conduction is blocked so that the ventricular rate is slowed. The atrial activity becomes obvious, which helps to identify the rhythm. Carotid sinus pressure seldom converts atrial flutter to sinus rhythm.

CSP AND ATRIAL FLUTTER

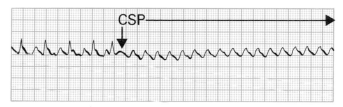

Note: Carotid sinus pressure increases the block at the AV node. Ventricular activity is completely suppressed and 'flutter' waves are obvious. Carotid sinus pressure can cause prolonged ventricular standstill and can produce a syncopal attack.

In atrial tachycardia, and *junctional tachycardia,* carotid sinus pressure may restore sinus rhythm.

CSP AND JUNCTIONAL TACHYCARDIA

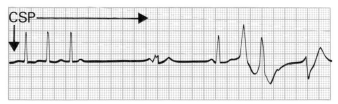

Note: Carotid sinus pressure reverts junctional tachycardia to sinus rhythm, but in this case multifocal ventricular extrasystoles occurred. Carotid sinus pressure should only be performed while the ECG is being monitored.

In atrial fibrillation and *ventricular tachycardia,* carotid sinus pressure has no effect, and with these or any other rhythms drug therapy may be needed.

Supraventricular tachycardias

(a) *Sinus tachycardia.* Sinus tachycardia is a response to pain, anxiety, hypovolaemia, thyrotoxicosis, anaemia, pregnancy, CO_2 retention, phaeochromocytoma, or treatment with beta-agonist drugs. It is the primary cause which should be treated, not the sinus tachycardia itself.

(b) *Junctional tachycardia*
    Carotid sinus massage
    Verapamil 5–10 mg i.v.

OR Practolol 5 mg i.v. repeated at 5 min intervals to 20 mg.

N.B. These two drugs should not be administered together, and Verapamil should not be given to patients on a beta blocker.
    DC shock.

Second line drugs: digoxin, disopyramide, amiodarone.

N.B. Unwanted effects of Verapamil may be reversed by calcium gluconate.

Prophylaxis for paroxysmal junctional tachycardia: try —
1. Digoxin
2. Propanolol
3. Verapamil
4. Disopyramide
5. Amiodarone

(c) *Atrial tachycardia.* N.B. May be due to digoxin toxicity. Treat as for junctional tachycardia.

(d) *Atrial fibrillation and flutter.* If the ventricular rate is less than 80 per minute no treatment is needed. For immediate control of a rapid ventricular rate give:

1. digoxin 250 micrograms i.v. slow injection at 30 min intervals to 1 mg.

OR

2. Practolol 5 mg i.v. repeated at 5 min intervals to 20 mg.

3. Amiodarone (dose as for VT — see below).

N.B. Amiodarone can potentiate digitalis effect.
If cardioversion is needed in a digitalised patient begin with very low energy shocks.

Most patients who develop AF after an MI will revert to sinus rhythm, but AF is a bad prognostic sign. Atrial flutter can be difficult to control, and cardioversion or atrial overdrive pacing may be needed.

For routine digitalisation, digoxin orally 500 micrograms initially followed by 250 micrograms tds for 2 days. The maintenance dose of digoxin depends on the patient's renal function. 125–250 micrograms daily is usually adequate; old people and those with renal failure may need 62.5 micrograms daily.

N.B. Hypokalaemia potentiates digoxin effects.

Ventricular tachycardia (broad complex tachycardia rate ⩾120/min)

1. Lignocaine 100 mg i.v. repeated at 5 min intervals × 2 followed by lignocaine infusion at 2–3 mg/min.
   N.B. Lignocaine causes hypotension, drowsiness, and sometimes fits.

2. Practolol 5 mg i.v. repeated at 5 minute intervals to 20 mg.

3. Flecainide 50–100 mg i.v.; for long term treatment 100 mg b.d. by mouth.
4. Amiodarone 300 mg in 250 ml dextrose over 30 min then 900 mg in 500 ml over 24 hours, followed by 200 mg t.d.s. by mouth for one week, followed by 200 mg b.d. for one week and 200 mg daily thereafter.

   N.B. Amiodarone must be given into a deep vein by long line. Ovedose prolongs Q.T. interval and can cause tachycardia. Long term treatment with amiodarone may cause skin pigmentation, photosensitive rashes, abnormalities of thyroid function, drug deposits in the cornea, and occasionally pulmonary fibrosis.

Second line drugs: disopyramide, mexilitine. Recurrent episodes of ventricular tachycardia, particularly those that are drug-induced, can be terminated and sometimes prevented by pacing the right ventricle with a temporary pacemaker. In 'overdrive' pacing the rate is set faster than that of the VT, and once the rhythm is captured by the pacemaker the rate can be slowed. Recurrent VT may be prevented by pacing at a rate of about 100 per minute.

Wolff-Parkinson-White Syndrome

For tachycardias associated with WPW:
1. IV Verapamil 5–10 mg i.v. (not if patient is on a beta blocker).

OR

   Practolol 5 mg i.v. repeated to 20 mg.
2. Flecainide
3. Amiodarone

For prophylaxis against paroxysmal arrhythmias try:
(1) Propanolol; (2) Flecainide; and (3) Amiodarone.

Bradycardias

Bradycardias must be treated if they are associated with hypotension, poor peripheral perfusion, or escape arrhythmias.

Any bradycardia can be treated with:

1. Atropine 600 micrograms i.v. repeated if necessary at 5 min intervals to 1.8 mg.
   N.B. Overdose causes tachycardia, hallucinations and urinary retention.
2. Isoprenaline 1–4 micrograms per min (2 mg in 500 ml dextrose = 4 micrograms per ml)
   N.B. Overdose causes ventricular arrhythmias which can be difficult to treat. An isoprenaline infusion should only be used while preparations are made for pacing.

Temporary pacing in patients with acute myocardial infarction. Pacing *should* be performed under the following circumstances:

1. Complete block with ventricular rate below 50 per minute.
2. Complete block with anterior infarction.
3. Any persistent bradycardia needing an isoprenaline infusion.
4. Bifascicular block plus first degree block.

Pacing should be *considered* for:

1. Any complete block.
2. Second degree block with heart rate less than 50 per min.
3. Bundle branch block plus first degree block.
4. Evidence of increasing block.
5. Bradycardia with escape rhythms.
6. For the treatment of tachyarrhythmias induced by drugs such as lidoflazine, quinidine etc.

Pacing is not necessary for:
1. First degree block.
2. Second degree block with ventricular rate over 50 per min.
3. Bundle branch block.

Permanent pacing. Insertion of a permanent pacemaker should be considered in a patient with complete heart block due to myocardial infarction who has had a temporary pacemaker for more than a week (remember that 95% of patients who develop complete block after myocardial infarction eventually regain sinus rhythm).

The prognosis of chronic complete heart block is relatively poor: if the patient has symptoms the mortality is 25–50% in the first year. The prognosis is improved by the insertion of a permanent pacemaker, and permanent pacing is indicated in patients of any age who have symptoms due to any persistent or intermittent bradycardia.

Chapter 3
The ECG in patients with chest pain

History and examination

The most important causes of acute chest pain are myocardial infarction, pulmonary embolism, pleuritic pain due to conditions other than embolism, pericarditis, dissection of the aorta, rupture or inflammation of the oesophagus, and collapse of a vertebra with root pain. All the non-cardiac conditions can mimic a myocardial infarction, and the ECG can be extremely useful for making a diagnosis of infarction. However, the ECG is less important than the history and physical examination for it can be normal in the first few hours of a myocardial infarction.

Acute chest pain

The pain of myocardial infarction is typically in the centre of the front of the chest, and it may radiate to the neck, jaw, teeth, arms, or back. It is often severe, and is then associated with sweating and sometimes vomiting. However, the pain can be mild or even occasionally absent.

The pain of a large central pulmonary embolus can be similar to that of myocardial infarction, but breathlessness and dizziness are usually also present. A peripheral pulmonary embolus will cause pleuritic pain and haemoptysis and pleuritic pain is usually easy to identify from the effect of respiration and coughing. Pericardial pain is usually worse lying flat and is relieved by sitting up and leaning forward; it may be affected by inspiration. The pain of aortic dissection is often described by the patient as 'tearing' (as opposed to the 'crushing' pain of myocardial infarction) and it is typically mainly felt in the back. Oesophageal rupture is always preceded by vomiting, and other oesophageal pain is usually associated with food and is typically worse on lying down. Pain due to spinal disease can be identified from the effect of movement and position.

In all these conditions the physical examination may be dominated by the effect of the pain itself: the patient may be anxious, often restless, and may be cold and sweaty. He will usually have a sinus tachycardia. The blood pressure is obviously important but diagnostically not necessarily helpful, for it can be low due to failure of the heart as a pump, or high due to intense peripheral vasoconstriction.

Each condition that causes chest pain may be associated with specific physical signs that are virtually diagnostic, but in each case these may be absent and this is particularly likely in the early stages of the illness.

In myocardial infarction there may be pulmonary oedema and the jugular venous pulse may be elevated; there may be a third or fourth heart sound at the cardiac apex. A large central pulmonary embolus will usually cause cyanosis and elevation of the jugular venous pressure, but there will be no added sounds in the lungs. Pleuritic pain of any cause, and also pericarditis, will be associated with a friction rub. Aortic dissection may cause the appearance of aortic valve regurgitation, and peripheral pulses may be lost; if blood tracks back to the pericardium there may be a pericardial friction rub. Vertebral collapse usually causes local tenderness. Oesophageal rupture causes few specific signs and is a very easy diagnosis to miss.

As usual in medicine, the history is more helpful in the diagnosis of chest pain than the physical examination, and both are more important than the ECG in the early stages of the patient's illness.

Chronic chest pain

The commonest causes of chronic or intermittent chest pain are angina and musculo-skeletal pain. An accurate diagnosis depends very much on the history: central crushing chest pain that radiates to the neck, jaw or teeth, or to the arm, and which is induced by exercise and is relieved by rest, is likely to be angina. Typically the pain is worse in cold or windy weather, or during exercise after a meal; it is induced by sexual intercourse and also by excitement or emotional stress. Angina is often accompanied by breathlessness. Pain that has similar characteristics but which is not closely related to exercise may be due to spasm of the coronary arteries, but much more often such pain is 'non-specific chest pain'. This sort of pain is common in young and middle aged men. It is usually felt in the left side of the chest and may radiate to the left arm. It commonly occurs after exercise, or at the end of a busy day, and it may last an hour or more. Although it may apparently be induced by emotional stress it is never caused by sexual intercourse.

Although angina is most often due to coronary artery disease it is important to remember that it may be due to an arrhythmia, hypertension, valve disease (especially aortic valve disease), to a cardiomyopathy, and to anaemia. It is important to exclude these possibilities by physical examination. Coronary artery disease itself causes no physical abnormalities but a previous infarction may cause an enlarged heart, heart failure, and perhaps mitral regurgitation. The signs of peripheral vascular disease may provide circumstantial evidence for the presence of coronary disease.

Non-specific chest pain causes no helpful abnormal signs, though chest wall tenderness may be present.

The ECG in patients with chest pain

Only after a full history has been taken and a careful physical examination has been made is it sensible to look at the ECG. The ECG is helpful when it shows unequivocal abnormalities, but when it does not it is much safer to rely on the patient's history and physical signs to make the diagnosis.

Among the various conditions that cause chest pain, the ECG is most useful in the diagnosis of myocardial infarction. It is helpful in the diagnosis of angina if a recording can be made when the patient has pain. It may provide confirmatory evidence of a pulmonary embolus but the changes are seldom diagnostic, and although in pericarditis there may be

ECG abnormalities these are usually non specific and the ECG is not often very helpful.

The ECG in myocardial infarction

It must be remembered that 'myocardial infarction' is really a pathological diagnosis, and if the patient survives there is no certain way of confirming that an infarction has occurred. There has been much disagreement about a clinical definition for myocardial infarction: when the story is clear, the ECG unequivocal and the serum enzymes that correlate with infarction (aspartate transaminase and lactate dehydrogenase) rise to twice their upper limit of normal then there will be little doubt that infarction has occurred. However, it can be difficult to be certain that ECG changes are new, and a marginal rise of serum enzymes is common in patients with suspected infarction. It is best only to label the patient as having had a 'definite' infarction when *both* the ECG and the serum enzymes show unequivocal changes, and where one of these is doubtful 'probable infarction' is an acceptable diagnosis. When neither is unequivocal 'possible infarction' is a reasonable label, but this merges into 'ischaemic disease without evidence of infarction'. 'Chest pain, ? cause' is an entirely proper diagnosis when the ECG and the serum enzymes are normal but the patient is admitted with chest pain for which no diagnosis can be made.

The development of ECG changes in infarction. The most important function of the ECG in patients with suspected myocardial infarction is to monitor the rhythm of the heart so that significant arrhythmias (especially ventricular fibrillation) can be treated rapidly. Rhythm problems have been considered in Chapter 2, and here we need to think about the ECG as a diagnostic aid.

It is essential to remember that in the first hour or more after the onset of chest pain due to myocardial infarction the ECG can remain normal. Up to 20% of patients admitted to hospital with what subsequently proves to be a myocardial infarction may show little or no abnormality in their first ECG. On the other hand, fully developed infarct patterns can be present very quickly indeed. Typically the ST segment first becomes raised, then Q waves appear, and finally the ST segment returns to the baseline and the T waves become inverted.

DEVELOPMENT OF INFERIOR MYOCARDIAL INFARCTION

	I	II	III	VR	VL	VF
Time from onset 30 min						
2 h						
24 h						
48 h						
72 h						

Note: Initial ECG shows inverted T in VL but no other abnormality.

ST segment then becomes elevated in the inferior leads.

Q waves develop, the ST segment returns to normal, and the T waves become inverted.

Because there is a very variable speed of development of the ECG changes in myocardial infarction it is difficult to decide from a single ECG when the infarction occurred. Serial changes in 2 or 3 records taken in the first three days of a suspected infarction are the most convincing evidence. Although classically the raised ST segment returns to the ECG baseline this does not always occur, and particularly with anterior infarction a raised ST segment may persist indefinitely. This is sometimes associated with a left ventricular aneurysm, but it is not a reliable way of making this diagnosis.

OLD ANTERIOR INFARCTION: LEFT VENTRICULAR ANEURYSM

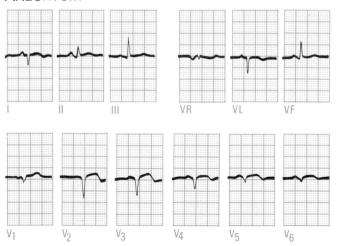

Note: This patient had an anterior infarction several months previously, but the ST segments in leads V_2–V_5 remain elevated. In this case a left ventricular aneurysm was present.

Once present, Q waves usually persist but when the infarction is small Q waves can disappear over a period of months and the ECG can return to normal. When this happens the patient's prognosis is very good.

The part of the heart that is infarcted is indicated by the ECG leads that show the infarct pattern. Thus an infarction of the anterior wall of the left ventricle and the septum causes changes in the leads that 'look at' the front of the heart, V_2–V_5.

ANTERIOR INFARCTION

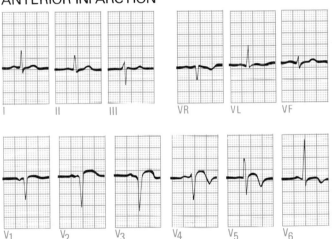

Note: The ECG is normal in the limb leads apart from T wave flattening in VL.

There is a Q in V_1–V_3 and only a rudimentary R in V_4.

The ST segment is elevated in V_2–V_5.

The T is inverted in V_4–V_6.

When the infarction affects the anterior and lateral wall of the left ventricle the changes occur in the anterior leads and also in the leads that 'look at' the lateral aspect of the heart, namely 1, VL, and V_5–V_6.

ACUTE ANTERO-LATERAL INFARCTION

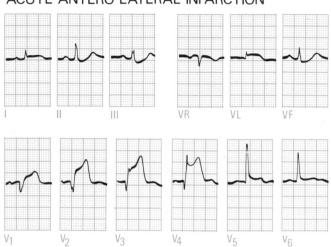

Note: Raised ST segments in I, VL, and V_2—V_6.
Q waves in V_2 to V_4.

When the inferior wall of the left ventricle is affected the ECG changes are seen in the 'inferior' leads, III and VF, and sometimes also in lead II.

INFERIOR INFARCTION

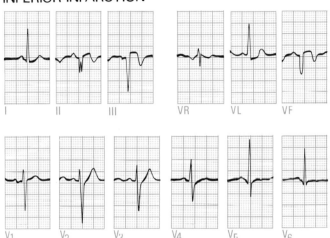

Note: Q waves with raised ST segment and inverted T waves in leads II, III and VF.
The chest leads show a normal appearance.

Infarction of both the anterior and inferior walls of the left ventricle cause changes in both the anterior and the inferior leads.

ANTERIOR AND INFERIOR INFARCTION

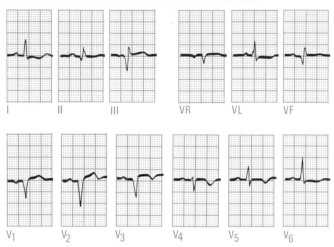

Note: Q waves in III and VF indicate old inferior infarction.
Q waves in V_2 and V_3, and a rudimentary R wave in V_4, plus inverted T waves in VL and V_3—V_6 indicate an anterior infarction and lateral ischaemia.

It is possible to 'look at' the back of the heart by placing the V lead on the back of the left side of the chest, but this is not done routinely as it is inconvenient, and the complexes recorded are often small. An infarction of the posterior wall of the left ventricle is, however, more easily detected in the ordinary 12 lead ECG because it causes a dominant R wave in lead V_1. The shape of the QRS complex recorded by V_1 depends on the balance of electrical forces under the ECG electrode. Normally the right ventricle is being depolarised towards this electrode, so causing an upward movement (an R wave) in the recording, and at the same time the posterior wall of the left ventricle is being depolarised with the wave of excitation moving away from the electrode and so causing a downward movement (an S wave) in the record. The left ventricle is more muscular than the right and it exerts a greater influence on the ECG, so in V_1 the QRS complex is predominantly downward (ie, there is a small R wave and a deep S). In a posterior infarction the rearward moving forces are lost, so V_1 'sees' the unopposed forward moving depolarisation of the right ventricle and records a predominantly upright QRS.

POSTERIOR INFARCTION

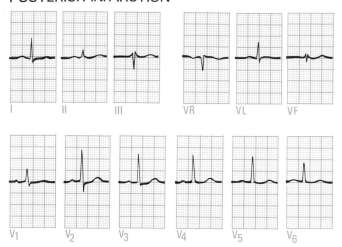

Note: The limb leads are normal.
 In V_1 there is a dominant R wave.
 There are no other changes to suggest right
 ventricular hypertrophy.

A posterior infarction is sometimes called a 'true posterior' infarction, because in old terminology what is now called 'inferior' used to be called 'posterior'. The dominant R wave of a (true) posterior infarction causes an ECG appearance very similar to that of right ventricular hypertrophy, but there is no accompanying right axis deviation. It is, however, the patient's history and the lack of right ventricular hypertrophy on physical examination that are most important in making the diagnosis.

Infarction can affect both the posterior and lateral walls of the left ventricle.

POSTERO-LATERAL INFARCTION

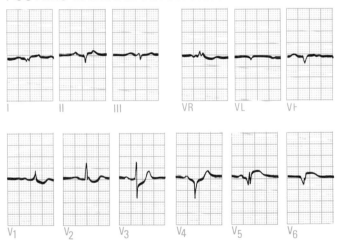

Note: Sinus rhythm.
Dominant R wave in V_1.
Q waves in I, VL, V_5—V_6 elevated ST segments in VL and V_5—V_6.

When a patient has a second myocardial infarction the ECG will show whether a second part of the left ventricle has been damaged. The next three ECGs show how useful sequential recordings can be.

1st RECORD: INFERIOR INFARCTION

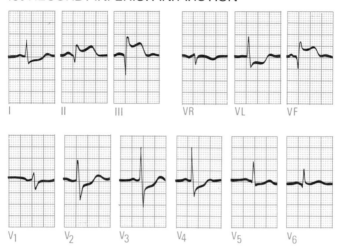

Note: This record was taken from a patient with recent onset of chest pain, and shows an acute inferior infarction with Q waves and raised ST segments in leads II, III and VF, plus ischaemic ST segment depression (see below) in the anterior leads.

Subsequently the patient had more pain.

2nd RECORD: AF, INFERIOR AND ANTERIOR INFARCTION

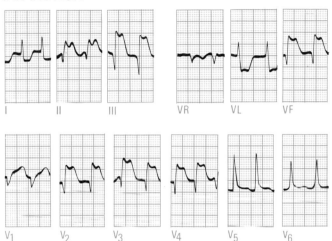

Note: This record shows atrial fibrillation with a rapid ventricular rate. The chest leads now show a raised ST segment suggesting an acute anterior infarction.

The patient recovered and sinus rhythm was restored.

3rd RECORD: SR, INFERIOR AND ANTERIOR INFARCTION

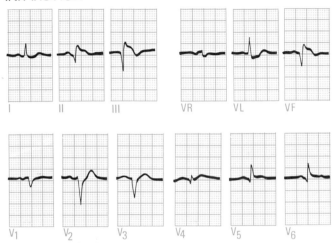

Note: Sinus rhythm
The ECG now shows a loss of R waves in V_2–V_4 and a diagnosis of both inferior and anterior infarction can be made.

A few weeks later the patient's ECG showed evidence of an old inferior and an old anterior infarction.

4th RECORD: OLD INFERIOR AND ANTERIOR INFARCTION

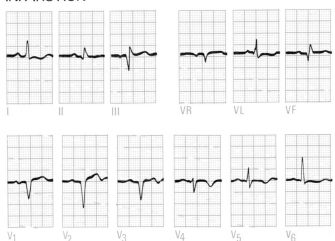

Note: In the inferior leads III and VF the Q waves persist but the T waves have become upright. Q waves in V_2–V_3 and inverted T waves in V_3–V_6 show an old anterior infarction.

A large infarction of the interventricular septum can cause damage to both bundle branches, and the ECG pattern of combined right and left bundle branch block is, of course, complete heart block. The QRS complex is then wide and the T wave abnormal, and no infarct pattern can be detected. Similarly, if an infarction causes left bundle branch block it is not possible to detect infarct changes on the ECG.

LEFT BUNDLE BRANCH BLOCK

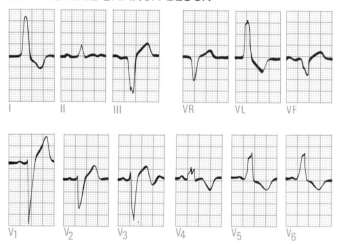

I   II   III   VR   VL   VF

V_1 V_2 V_3 V_4 V_5 V_6

Note: Sinus rhythm.
Broad QRS complexes with a notched R wave in V_5–V_6 show LBBB.
Inverted T waves are associated with LBBB.
Any ischaemia is masked by this pattern.

However, block of only the anterior fascicle of the left bundle branch does not obscure the infarction pattern, and the pattern of marked left axis deviation (left anterior hemiblock — see Ch. 6) and an anterior infarction pattern shows that part of the septum has been damaged.

LEFT ANTERIOR HEMIBLOCK WITH ANTERIOR INFARCTION

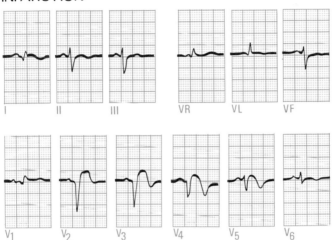

Note: Sinus rhythm.

Deep S waves in leads II and III show left axis deviation.

Anterior chest leads show elevated ST segment and inverted T waves due to anterior infarction.

With right bundle branch block due to septal infarction it is sometimes possible to be confident that an infarction has occurred.

RBBB WITH ANTERIOR INFARCTION

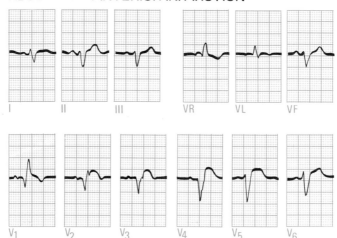

Note: Sinus rhythm.
RSR pattern in V_1 shows RBBB.
Q waves in V_2–V_4 with raised ST segments show anterior infarction.

Subendocardial infarction. When the infarction
does not involve the whole thickness of the
ventricular wall no electrical 'window' will be formed,
so there will be no Q waves. There will, however, be
an abnormality of repolarisation that leads to
inversion of the T waves. This pattern is sometimes
called 'subendocardial infarction', and it is most
commonly seen in the anterior and lateral leads.

SUBENDOCARDIAL INFARCTION

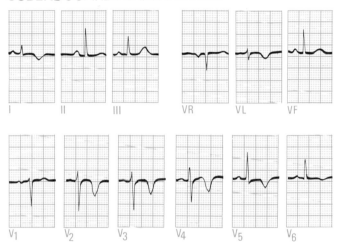

Note: No Q waves are present but the T waves are
inverted in I, VL, and V_2–V_6 due to
anterolateral subendocardial infarction.

It is important to remember that there are other causes of T inversion — and particularly that right ventricular hypertrophy causes T inversion in V_1 and V_2 (and sometimes in V_3) while left ventricular hypertrophy causes T inversion in I, VL, and V_6. The T wave inversion associated with the Wolff-Parkinson-White syndrome can at first sight cause a mistaken diagnosis of subendocardial infarction.

WOLFF-PARKINSON-WHITE SYNDROME

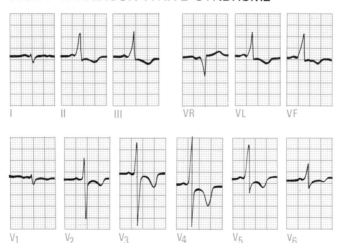

Note: Sinus rhythm with a short PR interval and slurred upstroke of the R wave due to pre-excitation.
Inverted T waves V_2–V_5 are characteristic of WPW and must not be mistaken for a subendocardial infarction.

In hypertrophic cardiomyopathy (a condition that may present with ischaemic cardiac pain) the ECG may show widespread deep T wave inversion resembling a subendocardial infarction.

HYPERTROPHIC CARDIOMYOPATHY

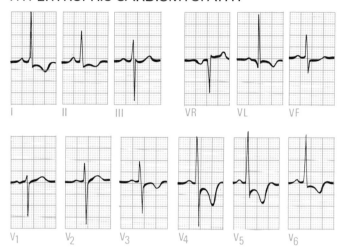

Note: Marked T wave inversion in the anterolateral leads, giving an appearance more like ischaemia than left ventricular hypertrophy.

The ECG in patients with angina

The patient who has angina but who has not had a myocardial infarction will usually have a normal ECG while he is free of pain. The ECG will become abnormal when the patient has angina, and the characteristic change is horizontal depression of the ST segment.

ISCHAEMIA

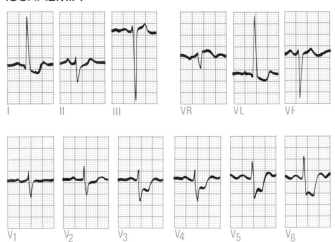

Note: Sinus rhythm with left axis deviation. Horizontal depression of the ST segments in leads V_3–V_6 indicates ischaemia.

The diagnosis of ischaemic pain can be made whatever the precipitating cause, and for example when pain occurs during a spontaneous episode of a paroxysmal attack of supraventricular tachycardia, depression in the ST segment indicates ischaemia.

ISCHAEMIA DURING JUNCTIONAL TACHYCARDIA

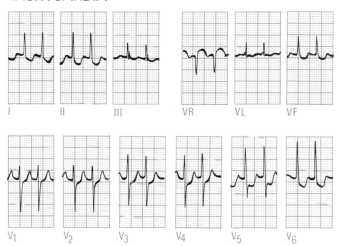

Note: Junctional tachycardia (no P waves and narrow QRS complexes) at 170 per min. ST segment depression in I, II, V_3–V_6 indicates ischaemia.

Angina can occur at rest due to spasm of the coronary arteries. This is accompanied by elevation rather than depression of the ST segment. The ECG appearance is similar to that of an acute myocardial infarction, but the ST segment returns to normal as the pain settles. This ECG appearance was first described by Prinzmetal, and it is sometimes called 'variant' angina.

PRINZMETAL'S VARIANT ANGINA

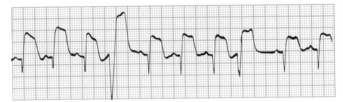

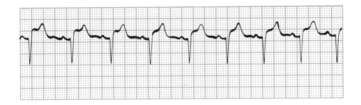

Note: The two strips form a continuous record. Initially the ST segment is raised; the fourth beat is probably a ventricular extrasystole. The ST segment quickly settles towards normal.

In most patients with intermittent chest pain, however, it will be necessary to stress the patient in some way to induce angina, and the safest procedure for this is the exercise test.

Exercise testing

Although any form of exercise that induces pain should produce ischaemic changes in the ECG, it is best to use a reproducible test that patients find relatively easy to perform, and to use carefully graded increments of exercise. The use of non-standard tests means that their results may be difficult to interpret, and particularly that repeated tests in the same patient cannot be compared. It is important to remember that changes in the ST segment of the ECG are only one piece of information that exercise provides, and the test should also be used to study the pumping action of the heart and to see whether exercise induces arrhythmia.

Reproducible exercise testing requires either a bicycle ergometer or a treadmill. In either case the exercise should begin at a low level that the patient finds easy, and it should be made progressively more difficult. On a bicycle the pedal speed should be kept constant and the workload increased in 25 watt steps; on a treadmill both the slope and the speed can be changed and the protocol evolved by Bruce is the one most commonly used.

Table 3.1 Bruce protocol for treadmill testing. Three minutes at each stage

	Low level			Ordinary level				
Stage	01	02	03	1	2	3	4	5
Speed km/hour	2.7	2.7	2.7	2.7	4.0	5.5	6.8	8.0
Slope°	0	1.3	2.6	4.3	5.4	6.3	7.2	8.1

A 12 lead ECG, the heart rate and the blood pressure should be recorded at the end of each 3 minute exercise period. Indications for discontinuing the test are:

1. At the request of the patient because of pain, breathlessness, fatigue, or dizziness.
2. If the systolic blood pressure begins to fall. Normally systolic pressure will rise progressively with increasing exercise levels, but in any subject a point will be reached when systolic pressure plateaus and then starts to fall. A fall of 10 mmHg is an indication that the heart is not pumping effectively, and the test should be stopped; if it is continued the patient will become dizzy and may fall. In healthy subjects a fall in systolic pressure is only seen at high work loads, but patients with severe heart disease may fail to elevate their systolic pressure on exercise. The amount of exercise the patient can achieve before the systolic pressure falls is thus a useful index of the severity of heart disease.
3. It is conventional to discontinue the test if the heart rate increases to 80% of the predicted maximum for the patient's age: this maximum can be calculated as 220 minus the patient's age in years. Patients with severe heart disease will usually fail

to attain 80% of their predicted maximum heart rate, and so the peak heart rate achieved is another useful indicator of the state of the patient's heart. It is, of course, important to take note of any treatment the patient may be receiving, for a beta blocker will prevent the normal heart rate increase. The maximum heart rate and blood pressure are in some ways more important than the maximum workload achieved because this is markedly influenced by physical fitness.

4. Exercise should be discontinued immediately if an arrhythmia occurs. The use of exercise testing to provoke arrhythmias is discussed in Chapter 2; many patients will have ventricular extrasystoles during exercise and these can be ignored unless their frequency begins to rise, or if a couplet of extrasystoles occurs.

5. The test should be stopped if the ST segment in any lead becomes depressed by 4 mm. 2 mm of horizontal depression in any lead constitutes a positive test, and if the aim of the test is to confirm or refute a diagnosis of angina there is no point in continuing once this has occurred. It may, however, be useful to find out just how much a patient can do, and if this is the aim it is not unreasonable to continue if the patient's symptoms are not severe.

The final report of the test should therefore indicate the duration of exercise and the workload achieved, the maximum heart rate and systolic pressure, the reason for discontinuing the test, and a description of any arrhythmias and ST segment changes.

Stage	Rest	02	1	2	3
Rate	95	123	131	148	168
BP	120/70	170/100	180/100	185/105	170/100

Note: Single complexes from each of leads V_0–V_6 at
rest and at then end of 4 stages of exercise on
the Bruce Protocol. Stage 02 is a low level of
exercise. With increasing exercise the heart
rate rises progressively, but at the final stage
the BP falls.

There is progressive ischaemic ST segment
depression in all leads but especially in V_4.

It is important to differentiate between ischaemic
changes in the ST segment and sloping ST or 'J
point' depression which is normal.

V_4 REST   EXERCISE

Note: Left hand complex is from V_4 at rest. Right
hand complex shows upward-sloping ST
segment during exercise, with depression of
the 'J' point.

This is a normal result.

Because exercise testing can induce arrhythmias it is necessary that the test should be supervised by a doctor.

REST

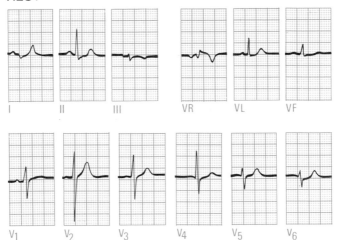

EXERCISE

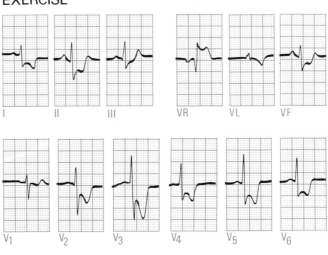

1 MINUTE AFTER EXERCISE

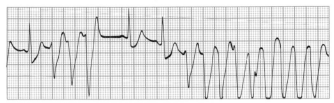

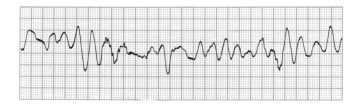

Note: Three records from a patient undergoing an
exercise test to establish a diagnosis of angina.
The record at rest is normal.
Exercise to the point when the patient
complained of chest pain caused marked
horizontal ST segment depression (8 mm in V_3)
with T inversion.
One minute after exercise there was a short
run of VT, followed by 2 sinus beats then a
return to VT which rapidly decayed to VF.

An alternative to a treadmill test, although usually less satisfactory, is to look for ST segment depression in an ambulatory ECG tape recording. It is important that the recorder is of the correct sensitivity for this test to be reliable. Ambulatory recording is mainly of value to study patients whose chest pain is not clearly related to exercise.

REST - NO PAIN

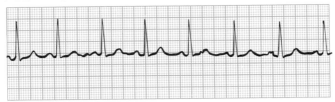

PAIN AT REST

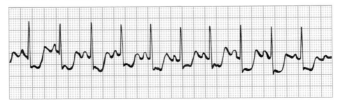

Note: Upper trace shows normal ECG in V_4. During an episode of chest pain at rest there is 4 mm ST segment depression.

The ECG in pulmonary embolism

Although the ECG can be helpful in making the diagnosis of pulmonary embolism it is not to be relied upon, for most patients with a pulmonary embolus will have no ECG abnormality other than a sinus tachycardia.

Pulmonary embolism causes problems for the right ventricle, and when multiple pulmonary emboli over a relatively long period cause chronic pulmonary hypertension the full range of changes due to right ventricular hypertrophy may be seen.

MULTIPLE PULMONARY EMBOLI

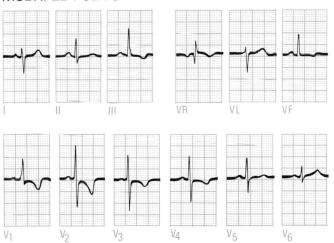

Note: Right axis deviation
Dominant R waves in V_1.
Persistent S waves in V_6.
Inverted T waves V_1–V_4.

It is, however, most unusual for the full ECG appearance of right ventricular hypertrophy to be seen with an acute pulmonary embolus. The diagnosis is likely if chest pain is associated with sinus tachycardia and any of these changes.

PULMONARY EMBOLUS

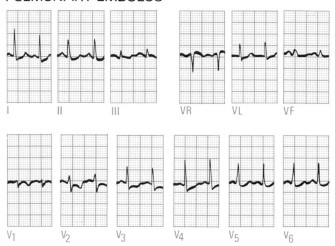

Note: Sinus tachycardia at 130 per min.
Normal QRS in V_1.
T inversion V_1–V_4.

In acute pulmonary embolism less dramatic changes will usually be seen. There may be isolated right axis deviation, but this can be a normal finding.

? PULMONARY EMBOLUS

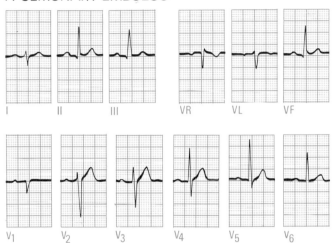

I   II   III   VR   VL   VF

V₁   V₂   V₃   V₄   V₅   V₆

Note: Dominant S in lead 1 indicates right axis deviation.
This could be normal, but it could also be the only ECG change due to a pulmonary embolus.

The significance of minor abnormalities may only be apparent if they are seen to appear in comparison with a previously normal ECG: for example, the appearance of T wave inversion in the right chest leads (V_1 and V_2) probably indicates a pulmonary embolus, though in a single ECG this appearance could be normal.

NORMAL ECG

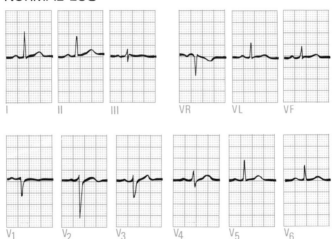

2 DAYS LATER: PULMONARY EMBOLUS

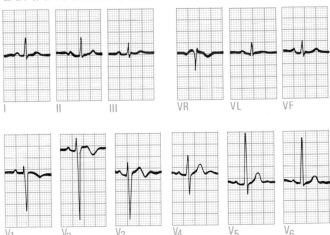

I   II   III   VR   VL   VF

V₁   V₂   V₃   V₄   V₅   V₆

Note: The first record (opposite) is entirely normal.
The second record (above), which was made 2
days later after an episode of chest pain,
shows T inversion in V_1 and V_2, and a biphasic
T in V_3. This record could be within normal
limits, but in comparison with the first it is
clearly abnormal and indicates a pulmonary
embolus. The change in height of the QRS
complex is not significant.

The combination of right axis deviation with a Q wave and an inverted T wave in lead III is said to be characteristic of pulmonary embolus, though it is by no means diagnostic.

PULMONARY EMBOLUS

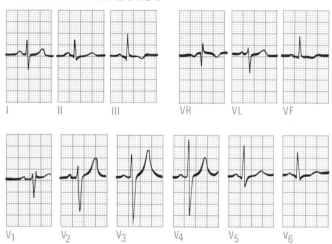

Note: 'S$_1$, Q$_3$, T$_3$' pattern of pulmonary embolus. The chest leads are normal.

Finally, acute pulmonary embolism may cause right bundle branch block, but again this is frequently seen in patients who do not have a pulmonary embolus so only the recorded appearance of this ECG abnormality is of much significance. Pulmonary emboli can also cause supraventricular arrhythmias.

PULMONARY EMBOLUS

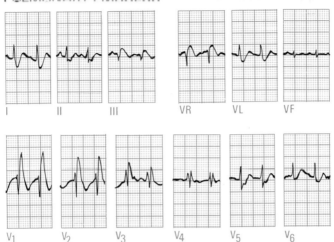

Note: Sinus tachycardia, rate 160 per minute.
Right bundle branch block.

The ECG in other causes of chest pain

Pericarditis may cause widespread ST/T changes. Classically the ST segment is elevated and the change resembles acute myocardial infarction with the difference that most leads are affected and Q waves do not develop. This 'classical' ECG pattern is in fact rare.

ACUTE PERICARDITIS

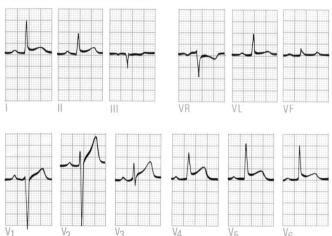

I   II   III   VR   VL   VF

V₁   V₂   V₃   V₄   V₅   V₆

Note: Widespread ST segment elevation, concave upwards.
No Q waves to suggest infarction.

If a patient complains of chest pain that sounds like
angina and the ECG shows left ventricular
hypertrophy it is important to remember that he may
have severe aortic valve disease and may need urgent
valve replacement.

LEFT VENTRICULAR HYPERTROPHY

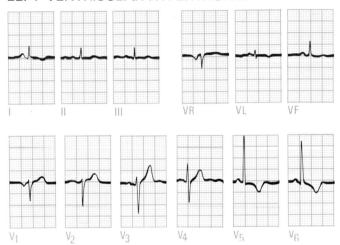

Note: Sinus rhythm with normal axis.
Tall R waves V_5–V_6.
Inverted T waves in 1, VL, V_5–V_6 indicate left
ventricular hypertrophy.

In patients with aortic dissection the ECG may show the changes of left ventricular hypertrophy if the patient has been hypertensive (see Ch. 4) but in many patients the dissection results from medial necrosis of the aorta without preceding hypertension, and the ECG is then normal. If the dissection occludes a coronary artery the ECG changes of an infarction may develop.

What to do

It is essential to remember that while the ECG can on occasions be extremely helpful in the diagnosis of chest pain, frequently it is not. The history, and to a lesser extent the physical examination, are far more important.

Acute chest pain

When a patient has a sudden attack of a new chest pain, the crucial decision is whether or not this could be due to a heart attack: this is one of the few conditions where making the right diagnosis and taking the right action can be lifesaving. If on clinical grounds a heart attack seems a reasonable possibility, the patient should be sent to hospital immediately unless the pain has been present for several hours, when the main risk of ventricular fibrillation will have passed. The distance the patient will have to travel, and the facilities available in the nearest hospital, will obviously influence the decision and so will the state of the patient: those with severe heart failure may well do better if allowed to respond to pain relief and diuretics before being subjected to a long ambulance journey.

Once in hospital the essential part of management is pain relief, which is best achieved with diamorphine or, if non-scheduled drugs are preferred, buprenorphine. The patient should be brought as quickly as possible to a place where the cardiac rhythm can be monitored and ventricular fibrillation treated with a defibrillator. He should *not* be sent for a chest X-ray, for this hardly ever helps in the management of the early stages of a heart attack; having a chest X-ray is taxing for a patient who is in pain and who feels ill, and it is often difficult to manage a cardiac arrest in an X-ray department.

When the patient has been admitted to a coronary care unit or ward detailed history taking and examination can be delayed until the pain has responded to treatment. No prophylactic antiarrhythmic treatment need be given. There is no need for the patient to stay in bed once he feels able to get up, and from the outset a positive and encouraging attitude must be taken about the prospects of early mobilisation, early discharge from hospital, and a rapid return to normality.

A chest X-ray is much more helpful if the history or physical examination suggest that the pain is pleuritic, and an X-ray is essential if a pneumothorax is possible. It may be difficult to distinguish infection from pulmonary embolism on a chest X-ray, and if in doubt there is little harm in giving heparin in addition to an antibiotic until the diagnosis is established. X-rays are also necessary if the history or physical signs suggest that the chest pain may be due to bone disease such as a collapsed thoracic vertebra causing root pain.

The most useful investigation when pericarditis is suspected is an echocardiogram. Pericarditis is usually associated with at least a small pericardial effusion, and this can readily be detected by echocardiography. It is, however, only necessary to perform this investigation as an emergency when there is evidence of cardiac tamponade. Blood investigations are seldom helpful in the acute phase of an illness with chest pain, though a sample should be taken for estimation of the white cell count and enzymes that rise with myocardial infarction (creatine kinase, aspartate transaminase, and lactate dehydrogenase).

Chronic or intermittent chest pain

If the patient's history suggests that chest pain is due to angina but the resting ECG is normal, it is worth performing an exercise test to establish the diagnosis. If from the history it is clear that the pain is non-specific it is not necessary to proceed to a time-consuming exercise test, though this can have a very useful therapeutic effect by demonstrating to the patient that his heart is normal. In neither case is the chest X-ray often helpful.

If the history suggests that the pain is oesophageal in origin a barium swallow X-ray or endoscopy is the appropriate investigation, but a therapeutic trial of antacids can be a useful and simple way of distinguishing oesophageal from cardiac pain. Both sorts of pain may respond to nitrates and calcium channel blockers, for these relieve oesophageal spasm.

Sublingual nitrates (glyceryl trinitrate 0.5 mg prn used prophylactically as well as when pain occurs) remain the mainstay of treatment for angina, though

any patient needing more than occasional nitrate
tablets should take continuously a beta blocker such
as atenolol 50–100 mg daily. If this proves ineffective
a calcium antagonist such as nifedipine (10–20 mg
tds) can be added, and so can a long-acting nitrate
(isosorbide dinitrate or mononitrate). If simultaneous
treatment with all 3 types of drug fails adequately to
control symptoms coronary angiography is necessary
to see whether coronary artery bypass grafting will be
helpful, and angiography should also be performed if
an exercise test reveals marked ischaemia at low
levels of workload.

Chapter 4
The ECG in patients with breathlessness

History and examination

Everyone is breathless at times, and people who are physically unfit or who are overweight will be more breathless than others. Breathlessness can also result from anxiety, but when it is due to physical illness the important causes are anaemia, heart disease, and lung disease; a combination of causes is common. The most important function of the history is to help decide whether the patient does indeed have a physical illness and if so, which system is at fault.

Breathlessness in heart disease is due either to increased lung stiffness as a result of pulmonary congestion, or to pulmonary oedema. Pulmonary congestion occurs when the left atrial pressure is high, which occurs either when mitral stenosis impairs blood flow from the left atrium to the left ventricle, or when the left ventricle is failing and its filling pressure (the end-diastolic pressure) is high. When the pressure within the pulmonary capillaries (which is the same as that in the pulmonary veins and left atrium) exceeds plasma oncotic pressure, fluid will leak into the alveoli and cause pulmonary oedema.

The presence of pulmonary oedema is relatively easy to recognise from the story of orthopnoea, severe breathlessness (especially with attacks at night) with wheeze and a cough productive of frothy sputum which may be pink or frankly blood stained. Physical examination reveals fine crackles over the lung bases and there are usually other signs of heart failure such as a raised jugular venous pressure, ankle swelling, or hepatic distension, and the heart is usually large.

The recognition of pulmonary congestion is less easy for it can be confused with chest disease causing right heart failure (cor pulmonale). In both the patient may complain of orthopnoea (breathlessness on lying flat): in heart failure this is due to the return of blood that was pooled in the legs to the effective circulation; in patients with chest disease (especially chronic obstructive airways disease) orthopnoea results from a need to use diaphragmatic respiration more effectively. Both pulmonary congestion and lung disease can cause a diffuse wheeze. Both pulmonary congestion and cor pulmonale will be associated with signs of right heart failure. The diagnosis therefore depends on a positive identification, either in the history or on examination, of heart or lung disease.

The main causes of heart failure are ischaemia, valve disease, hypertension, congenital defects, heart muscle disease, and arrhythmias. Ischaemia and arrhythmias can usually be suspected from the patient's symptoms and sometimes from the physical examination: the value of the ECG in diagnosing these conditions was considered in Chapters 2 and 3.

Congenital disease will be suspected from the history and examination, and the presence of valve disease may be suspected if the patient gives a history of previous rheumatic fever. However, the diagnosis of valve disease, heart muscle disease and hypertension depends mainly on the physical examination. The value of the ECG in these conditions is quite limited and in general all the ECG can do is to provide a limited amount of information about the size of the four heart chambers.

The ECG also has only limited value in the diagnosis of respiratory disease. The diagnosis depends on a history of cough, wheeze, and sputum production, and on the physical signs of lung disease. The ECG can only show whether sufficient lung disease is present to cause enlargement of the right atrium and right ventricle.

The ECG in disorders affecting the left side of the heart

The ECG in left atrial hypertrophy

Left atrial hypertrophy may be associated with left ventricular hypertrophy, but left atrial hypertrophy without left ventricular hypertrophy is virtually diagnostic of mitral stenosis. Mitral stenosis causes right ventricular hypertrophy and this may be evident on the ECG (see below). ECG evidence of left atrial hypertrophy is, however, seldom helpful in assessing the severity of mitral valve disease for most patients develop atrial fibrillation and with the loss of P waves no information about the size of the left atrium is available.

When the heart is in sinus rhythm, left atrial hypertrophy causes a broad and sometimes bifid P wave. Because this is characteristic of mitral stenosis this P wave abnormality is sometimes called 'P mitrale'.

LEFT ATRIAL HYPERTROPHY

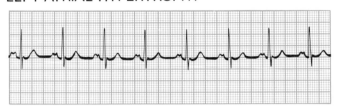

Note: Sinus rhythm.
        The P waves are broad and bifid (i.e. have 2 humps).

The ECG in left ventricular hypertrophy

Left ventricular hypertrophy may be caused by hypertension, aortic stenosis or incompetence, and mitral incompetence.

The electrocardiographic features of left ventricular hypertrophy are:
1. An increased height of the QRS complex.
2. Left axis deviation.
3. Inverted T waves in the leads that 'look at' the left ventricle — I, VL, and V_5–V_6.

Unfortunately, none of these features is an infallible indication of left ventricular size, and two records from patients with severe aortic stenosis illustrate the problem.

The first record, which was from a patient with congenital aortic stenosis with a pressure gradient across the valve of 80 mmHg (indicating severe stenosis) leaves no doubt about left ventricular hypertrophy.

LEFT VENTRICULAR HYPERTROPHY

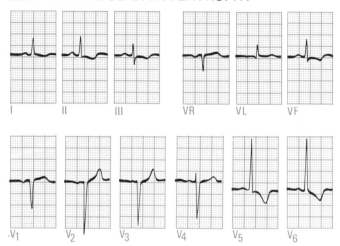

Note: Tall R wave in V_6 and deep S in V_2.
Inverted T waves in II, III, VF, V_5–V_6.
The axis is normal.

This appearance is sometimes referred to as a 'left ventricular strain' pattern, but this is a meaningless term. The record was in fact made 8 years after an aortic valve replacement, when the patient was completely well and the left ventricle was certainly not under 'strain', but the ECG appearance of left ventricular hypertrophy had not changed since before the operation.

The second record came from another patient with severe aortic stenosis (gradient of 85 mmHg across the valve) and the patient was breathless and needed valve replacement. The ECG was, however, entirely normal.

AORTIC STENOSIS: NORMAL RECORD

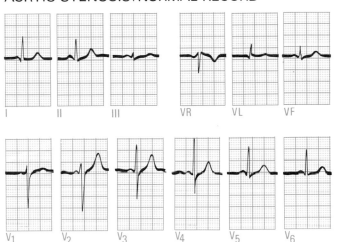

Note: No evidence of left ventricular hypertrophy. Normal sized QRS complexes and upright T waves.

Between these two extremes, ECG evidence of left ventricular hypertrophy can be very variable.

The normal maximum height of the R wave in lead V_5 or V_6, and also the normal maximum depth of the S wave in V_1 and V_2, is often set at 25 mm. The maximum height of the R in V_5 or V_6 plus the S in V_1

or V_2 is supposed in normal people to be less than 35 mm. However, these limits are frequently exceeded in the ECG of young fit people, particularly when they are thin (Ch. 1). The next ECG, however, came from an 18-year-old who had had an aortic valve replacement for congenital aortic stenosis.

? LEFT VENTRICULAR HYPERTROPHY

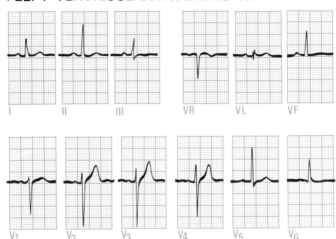

V leads at half sensitivity

Note: Sinus rhythm, normal axis.
The record looks entirely normal but the chest leads were recorded with a sensitivity 1mV = 0.5 cm. The 'true' height of the QRS complexes is thus twice what is recorded. The record shows LV hypertrophy by 'voltage' criteria.

As we have seen (Ch. 1) minor changes of left axis deviation occur in the ECGs of normal people who are short and fat. Marked left axis deviation may be seen in patients with left ventricular hypertrophy, but it is really an indication of a conduction defect rather than of ventricular mass. Marked left axis deviation is due to failure of conduction through the anterior fascicle of the left bundle branch ('left anterior hemiblock') and this can occur without any left ventricle enlargement.

The next ECG came from an asymptomatic patient whose heart was clinically normal.

LEFT ANTERIOR HEMIBLOCK

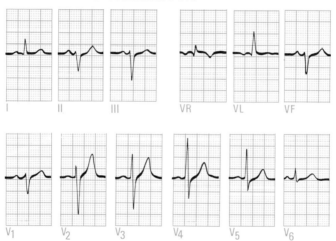

Note: Sinus rhythm.
Marked left axis deviation with a predominant S wave in leads II and III.

The combination of either tall complexes or left axis deviation with inverted T waves in the lateral leads makes a diagnosis of left ventricular hypertrophy likely, and in any patient with valvular disease the appearance of ECG changes of left ventricular hypertrophy in serial recordings should be taken as evidence of deterioration. However, the lateral T wave changes can vary from time to time, and the next record shows the chest leads in two records taken six months apart in an elderly patient with aortic valve disease.

LEFT VENTRICULAR HYPERTROPHY:
FIRST RECORD (chest leads only)

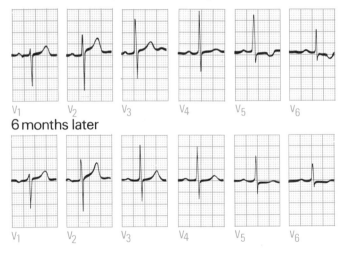

Note: First record (chest leads only) shows T inversion in V_5–V_6.
This is much less obvious in the second record.

Lateral T wave inversion can result from ischaemia as well as left ventricular hypertrophy, and the next record was from a patient with a myocardial infarction.

SUBENDOCARDIAL INFARCTION

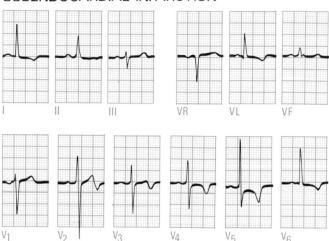

Note: Sinus rhythm, normal axis.
Normal QRS complexes.
T wave inversion V_2–V_6.

The presence of ischaemia rather than left ventricular hypertrophy should be suspected if any pathological Q waves are present, if T wave inversion is also present in the 'septal' lead V_4, or if T inversion is more marked in V_3–V_5 than in V_6.

The ECG in patients with conditions affecting the right side of the heart

The ECG in right atrial hypertrophy

Right atrial hypertrophy causes tall and peaked P waves. There is, in fact, such variation within the normal range of P waves that the diagnosis of right atrial hypertrophy is difficult to make, but its presence can be inferred when peaked P waves are associated with the ECG changes of right ventricular hypertrophy. The changes of right atrial hypertrophy without those of right ventricular hypertrophy will usually only be seen in patients with tricuspid stenosis.

RIGHT ATRIAL HYPERTROPHY

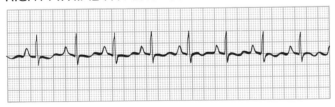

Note: Sinus rhythm.
Peaked P waves due to right atrial hypertrophy.
The T waves are inverted but in a single lead it is not possible to see why.

The ECG in right ventricular hypertrophy

The electrocardiographic changes associated with right ventricular hypertrophy are:

1. Right axis deviation.
2. A dominant R wave (i.e. the R wave height is greater than the S wave depth) in V_1.
3. 'Clockwise rotation' of the heart: as the right ventricle occupies more of the anterior surface of the chest and the septum is displaced laterally, the transition of the QRS complex in the chest leads from a right to a left ventricular configuration occurs in V_4–V_5 instead of V_2–V_3. There is thus a persistent S wave in lead V_6, which normally does not show an S wave at all.
4. Inversion of the T wave in leads that 'look at' the right ventricle — V_1 and V_2, and occasionally V_3.

In extreme cases it is easy to diagnose right ventricular hypertrophy from the ECG. The next record came from a patient incapacitated with breathlessness due to thromboembolic pulmonary hypertension.

SEVERE RIGHT VENTRICULAR HYPERTROPHY

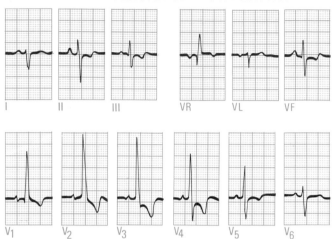

Note: Sinus rhythm with right axis deviation.
Dominant and very tall R wave in V_1–V_4.
R wave equals S wave (the 'transition point') in V_5.
Deep S wave in V_6.

However, as with the ECG in left ventricular hypertrophy, none of the changes on their own provide unequivocal evidence of right ventricular hypertrophy and conversely it is possible to have marked right ventricular hypertrophy without all the ECG features being present. Minor degrees of right axis deviation are seen in normal people and a dominant R wave in lead V_1 is occasionally seen in normal people although it is never more than 3 or 4 mm tall.

A dominant R in V_1 may also indicate a 'true posterior' myocardial infarction (see Ch. 3).

There is a marked variation in T wave Inversion in V_1 and V_2 in normal subjects (Ch. 1) and particularly in black people the T wave can be inverted in V_3. The next ECG was recorded from a young woman who claimed to be dizzy and breathless, and who might have had pulmonary hypertension. In fact her heart and lungs were entirely normal.

NORMAL ECG

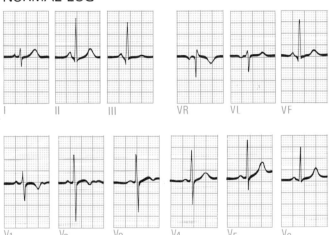

Note: Sinus rhythm with normal axis.
T wave inversion in V_1–V_2.
No other suggestion of right ventricular hypertrophy.

When the T wave inversion is more pronounced the ECG might be confused with a subendocardial infarction. The next record was from a young woman who did have thromboembolic pulmonary hypertension, and who was quite breathless.

RIGHT VENTRICULAR HYPERTROPHY

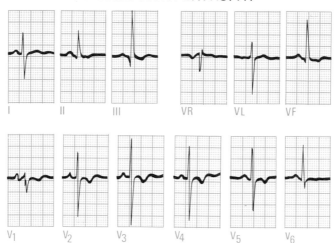

I   II   III   VR   VL   VF

V_1 V_2 V_3 V_4 V_5 V_6

Note: Sinus rhythm.
Dominant S wave in I shows right axis deviation, and this gives a clue to the cause of T wave inversion.
T inversion V_1–V_5.

When anterior T wave inversion is associated with both right axis deviation and a dominant R wave in V_1, the diagnosis becomes much more obvious and particularly so when T wave inversion is most marked in V_1 and gets progressively less marked in V_2 onwards.

RIGHT VENTRICULAR HYPERTROPHY

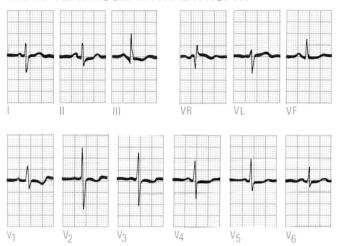

Note: Sinus rhythm.
Right axis deviation.
Dominant R in V_1.
T inversion V_1–V_4.

Marked 'clockwise rotation' can be a prominent feature of right ventricular hypertrophy.

RIGHT VENTRICULAR HYPERTROPHY

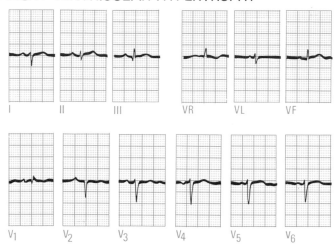

Note: Sinus rhythm with right axis deviation.
Small dominant R wave in V_1.
Marked 'clockwise rotation' of the heart with the right ventricle occupying the whole of the anterior surface of the heart. Even V_6 does not overly the septum. All the chest leads show a right ventricular complex.

An S wave in lead V_6, without other ECG evidence of right ventricular hypertrophy is characteristic of patients with chronic chest disease such as obstructive airways disease.

CHRONIC LUNG DISEASE

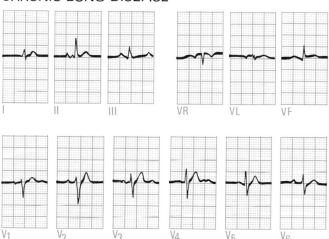

Note: The transition of the QRS complex from a right ventricular to a left ventricular type occurs in lead V_5, and there is an S wave in lead V_6. There is no other evidence of right ventricular hypertrophy.

As with the ECG in left ventricular hypertrophy, it is the appearance of changes in serial recordings that provides the best evidence of minor or moderate degrees of right ventricular hypertrophy.

In the majority of cases in which the ECG provides evidence of right ventricular hypertrophy it is not possible to diagnose the underlying disease process.

The exception to this is mitral stenosis, where obstruction to blood flow from the left atrium to the left ventricle causes left atrial hypertrophy, and provided the heart is in sinus rhythm this causes broad and bifid P waves. At the same time, raised pressure in the pulmonary veins causes pulmonary hypertension, and this in turn leads to right ventricular hypertrophy.

LA AND RV HYPERTROPHY IN MITRAL STENOSIS

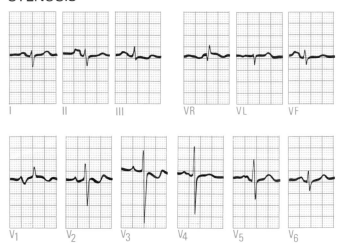

Note: Sinus rhythm with broad P waves due to left atrial hypertrophy.
Right axis deviation, a dominant R wave in V_1, inverted T waves V_1–V_3 and an S wave in V_6 indicate right ventricular hypertrophy.

The ECG in patients with congenital heart disease

The ECG provides a limited amount of help in the diagnosis of congenital heart disease by showing which chambers of the heart are enlarged. It is important to remember (Ch. 1) that at birth the ECG of a normal infant shows a pattern of 'right ventricular hypertrophy', and this gradually disappears in the first two years.

If the infant pattern persists beyond the age of 2, right ventricular hypertrophy is indeed present. If there is a left ventricular, or adult, pattern before this age then left ventricular hypertrophy is probably present. In older children the same criteria for left and right ventricular hypertrophy apply as in adults.

Table 4.1 lists the common congenital disorders and the associated ECG appearance.

Table 4.1 ECG appearance in the common congenital disorders

ECG	Congenital defect
Right ventricular hypertrophy	Pulmonary hypertension of any cause Severe pulmonary stenosis Fallot's tetralogy Transposition of the great arteries
Left ventricular hypertrophy	Aortic stenosis Coarctation of the aorta Mitral regurgitation Obstructive cardiomyopathy.
Biventricular hypertrophy	Ventricular septal defect
Right atrial hypertrophy	Tricuspid stenosis
Right bundle branch block	Atrial septal defect Complex defects.

RA AND RV HYPERTROPHY IN FALLOT'S TETRALOGY

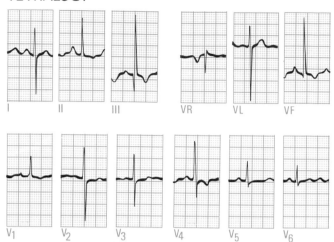

Note: Peaked P in lead II indicates right atrial hypertrophy.
Right axis deviation.
Dominant R in V_1 with inverted T in V_1–V_4. This trace shows the 'S$_1$, Q$_3$, T$_3$' pattern sometimes said to indicate pulmonary embolism, and shows that this combination is not diagnostic of any particular condition.

What to do

In most patients with breathlessness the ECG does not contribute very much to diagnosis and management, and the important thing is to treat the patient and not the ECG. The ECG cannot diagnose heart failure, although by demonstrating ischaemia or enlargement of one or more cardiac chambers it may help to elucidate the underlying disease that requires treatment. However, the symptoms of heart failure need empirical treatment whatever the ECG shows and this should not be delayed while an ECG is being recorded. Similarly, while the ECG can provide confirmatory evidence that breathlessness is due to a pulmonary embolus (Ch. 3) or chronic lung disease, it is an unreliable way of making this diagnosis and treatment cannot depend on the ECG. The ECG will not help the diagnosis of anaemia, though it may show ischaemic changes.

In general, then, the management of the breathless patient does not depend on the ECG but there are two important exceptions.

First, if breathlessness is due to heart failure which is secondary to an arrhythmia, then the ECG is essential both for diagnosis and for monitoring the response to therapy.

Second, the ECG has an important role in the timing of surgery for valve disease, and particularly for aortic valve disease. In aortic stenosis, left ventricular enlargement may not be obvious on examination even when the valve lesion is severe. Even in an asymptomatic patient the presence of left ventricular hypertrophy on the ECG is an indication for urgent cardiac catheterisation with a view to surgery, for when aortic stenosis is sufficiently severe to cause such changes the prognosis is poor. Serial recording of the ECG is one investigation that can be useful when monitoring the progress of patients with mitral and aortic valve disease, for the appearance of any changes will at least be a relative indication for surgery.

Chapter 5

The ECG as an aid to diagnosis

The ECG is not a good way to diagnose any condition that is not primarily cardiac in origin, but some generalised diseases involve the heart and cause ECG abnormalities. The value of the ECG is not so much to help make a diagnosis in such circumstances as to show that the heart has become involved in the disease process. It is also important to recognise some of the ECG abnormalities that general diseases can cause so that they are not confused with the changes of primary cardiac disease.

Artefacts in ECG recordings

Improper electrode placement

If the electrodes are wrongly attached to the limbs there will be abnormalities in the height of the P, QRS, and T waves, and the cardiac axis may seem bizarre; the ECG will, however, be normal in the V leads. When the P wave is upside down in leads other than AVR despite the patient being in sinus rhythm with a normal PR interval, or when the cardiac axis is difficult to calculate, improper electrode attachment should be suspected and the recording repeated.

NORMAL ECG ?

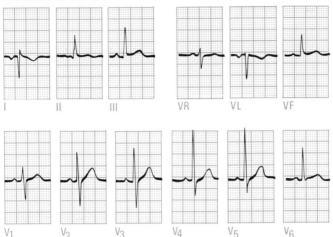

Note: In this ECG the right arm electrode has been
        attached to the left arm and vice versa. The P
        wave is upside down in leads I and VL. The
        appearance of the V leads is normal.

Dextrocardia causes similar abnormalities in the
standard leads to improper electrode attachment, but
the pattern of the chest leads is also abnormal. Leads
that normally 'look at' the left ventricle (V_5 and V_6)
record a 'right ventricular' complex (Ch. 1).

When an ECG appears odd it is always prudent to
suspect a technical error and repeat it.

NORMAL ECG?

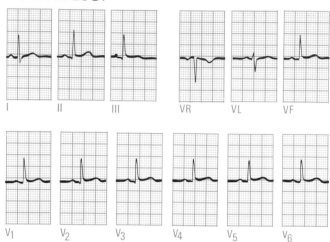

Note: The record in the standard leads is normal. In
all the 'chest leads' the QRS complex is
identical, and is the same as in VF. The 'chest
leads' have been recorded with the lead
selector left in the VF position.

The effects of abnormal muscle movement

The contraction of any muscle is initiated by a
depolarisation of the muscle cells, and although ECG
recorders are designed to be especially sensitive to
the frequencies of cardiac muscle the ECG will record
the contraction of skeletal muscle. The most common
pattern of 'ECG abnormality' is a high frequency
oscillation due to general muscular tension in a
patient who is not properly relaxed. This is
accentuated when the patient is cold and shivering.

HYPOTHERMIA

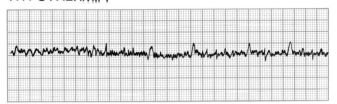

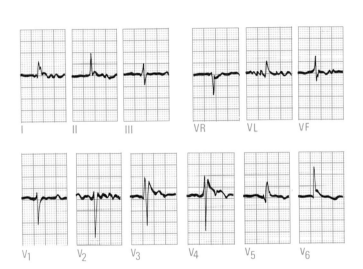

Note: Coarse 'muscle tremor' obscures any P waves that might be present, but the irregularity of the QRS complexes in the top strip suggests that the rhythm is atrial fibrillation.

In addition to the effect of generalised tremor the ECG of a hypothermic patient may show a hump (a J wave) at the end of the QRS complex. It is difficult to distinguish these in the above record. The J waves are clearly seen in the next record, which came from a hypothermic patient who was not shivering.

HYPOTHERMIA

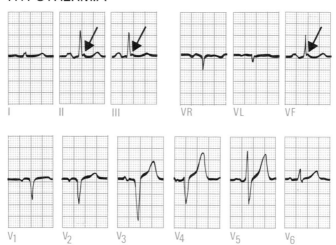

Note: The ECG is normal apart from 'J waves' at the end of the QRS complexes. These are most clearly seen in leads II, III and VF (arrows).

Sustained involuntary tremors cause rhythmic ECG abnormalities that may be confused with cardiac arrhythmias.

PARKINSONISM

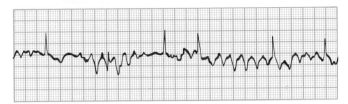

Note: Tremor at 5 per second gives an appearance
resembling atrial flutter. The patient was in
sinus rhythm but the QRS complexes appear
irregular, probably because of poor electrode
contact.

This record demonstrates the importance of
looking at the patient as well as the ECG.

The ECG in systemic diseases

Cardiac involvement in a generalised disorder, and
particularly those disorders that cause infiltration or
deposition of abnormal substances in the
myocardium, cause arrhythmias and conduction
defects.

Thyrotoxicosis is probably the most common
disorder that may present as a cardiac problem.
Particularly in old age there may be atrial fibrillation,
usually with a rapid ventricular response which is
difficult to control with Digoxin. An elderly patient
may complain mainly of palpitations or of the
symptoms of heart failure, and arterial embolisation
may occur; the usual symptoms of thyrotoxicosis
may be mild or even absent.

THYROTOXICOSIS

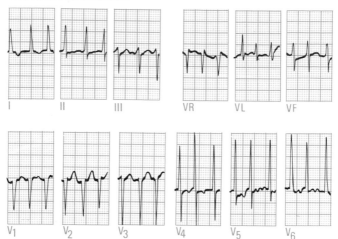

Note: Atrial fibrillation with a ventricular rate of
about 200 per minute.
The T waves are inverted in the anterior and
lateral leads, probably indicating ischaemia.

In *myxoedema* there will usually be a sinus
bradycardia and sometimes non-specific ST/T
changes; if there is a pericardial effusion the ECG
complexes may be small.
Malignant disease with cardiac secondary deposits
can cause atrial fibrillation, and a deposit
appropriately placed in the conducting system can
cause complete heart block. In Western countries
malignancy is the commonest cause of large
pericardial effusions (tuberculosis being more
common in underdeveloped countries) and the
combination of an arrhythmia with small complexes
suggests a mediastinal malignancy.

MALIGNANT PERICARDIAL EFFUSION

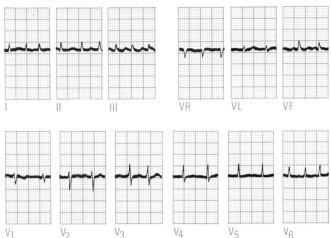

I   II   III   VR   VL   VF

V_1 V_2 V_3 V_4 V_5 V_6

Note: Atrial fibrillation with ventricular rate of about 150 per minute.
Small QRS complexes indicate pericardial effusion.

Electrolyte abnormalities

Hypokalaemia (most commonly the result of diuretic therapy) prolongs the QT interval, which is measured from the onset of the QRS complex to the end of the T wave. In hypokalaemia the T wave is flattened and is followed by a further low amplitude deflection called a U wave. U waves are commonly seen in normal records, particularly in the anterior chest leads V_2–V_4, but in a normal ECG the T wave is not flattened (Ch. 1). The next ECG was recorded from a patient with a serum potassium of 1.9 mmol/l.

HYPOKALAEMIA

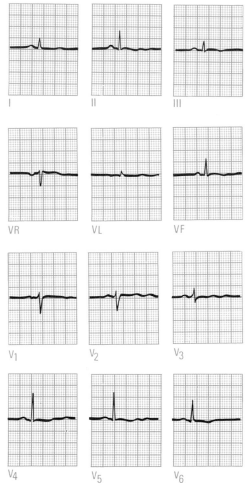

Note: Sinus rhythm with normal QRS complexes.
In all leads the T waves are flattened and it is
difficult to measure the QT interval, but this is
probably 0.44 seconds.
U waves are present in most leads.

The QT interval is also prolonged in hypocalcaemia and in severe rheumatic carditis.

Hyperkalaemia causes peaked T waves, but not much more than can be seen in normal ECGs (Ch. 1). The next ECG came from a patient with a serum potassium of 5.9 mmol/l.

HYPERKALAEMIA

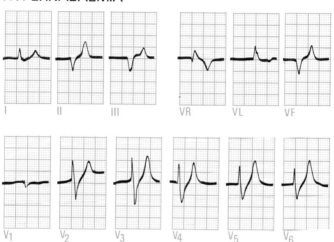

Note: Sinus rhythm with left axis deviation.
The T waves are peaked in all leads.

The effect of medication on the ECG

Digitalis

The main use of digoxin and the other drugs related to digitalis is to block atrioventricular conduction and so to slow the ventricular rate in atrial fibrillation. Provided A/V conduction is normal, atrial fibrillation will usually be associated with a rapid ventricular response, but a slow rate, particularly with regularity of the QRS complexes, suggests a digitalis effect. Digitalis also causes down-sloping depression of the ST segment with inversion of the T waves, and these changes are most pronounced in the left lateral lead (VL, V_5–V_6).

DIGITALIS EFFECT

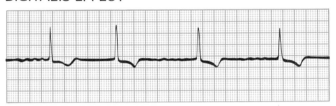

Note: Atrial fibrillation with a ventricular rate of about 50 per minute.
The ST segments slope downwards and the T waves are inverted, giving a 'reverse tick' appearance.

The effect of digoxin on the ECG must be differentiated from that of ischaemia, which causes horizontal ST segment depression. Both changes can sometimes be recognised in a single ECG.

ISCHAEMIA AND DIGOXIN

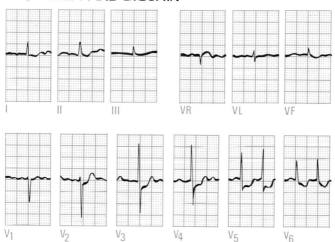

Note: Atrial fibrillation with a ventricular rate of 150 per minute at times.

In leads V_3–V_5 there is horizontal ST segment depression suggesting ischaemia. In V_6 the ST segment slopes downwards and the T wave is inverted; these changes are probably due to digoxin.

Digoxin toxicity causes almost any cardiac arrhythmia, including bradycardias and tachycardias. The most classical digoxin-induced arrhythmias are atrioventricular block, atrial tachycardia with block, and multifocal ventricular extrasystoles and sometimes ventricular tachycardia. These arrhythmias are particularly likely to occur in the presence of hypokalaemia.

DIGOXIN TOXICITY

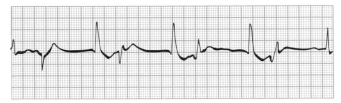

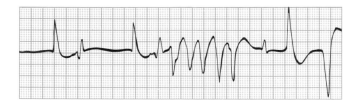

Note: The two strips form a continuous record. The basic rhythm is atrial fibrillation and the upright QRS complexes are probably the normally-conducted beats. Each of these is followed by a predominantly downward QRS, which represents a ventricular extrasystole. In the lower strip there is a short run of ventricular tachycardia.

Antiarrhythmic drugs

All the antiarrhythmic drugs of the 'class 1' type (quinidine, lignocaine, disopyramide, flecainide, etc) can all actually cause arrhythmias. Some prolong the QT interval (and amiodarone can also have this effect) but others do not; all cause ventricular tachycardia which is usually of the 'Torsade de pointes' type in which the QRS complexes change progressively due to changing re-entry pathways (Ch. 6).

Other drugs

Tricyclic antidepressants cause arrhythmias, and the antianginal drugs prenylamine and lidoflazine also cause 'Torsade' ventricular tachycardia.

PRENYLAMINE TOXICITY

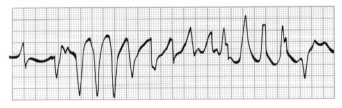

Note: A single sinus beat is followed by a run of ventricular tachycardia. The QRS complexes initially point downwards but then change progressively to an upright configuration. This writhing appearance is referred to as the 'Torsade de pointes' variety of ventricular tachycardia.

What to do

The ECG is a very unreliable aid to the diagnosis of problems in which the heart is only affected as part of an overall disease process. In most cases — for example in malignant disease — non-cardiac symptoms and signs will predominate, but in others (particularly thyrotoxicosis in the elderly) a cardiac abnormality may be the primary feature of the illness. As always in medicine, the first thing is not to place undue reliance on a single investigation, and second not to be satisfied with the immediate diagnosis. If the ECG reveals atrial fibrillation ask what is its cause. If the ECG raises the possibility of a pericardial effusion ask if this is consistent with the patient's appearance, and then think what a pericardial effusion could be due to. An ECG will define the nature of a conduction defect or an arrhythmia, but frequently will not indicate its cause, and the cause of the arrhythmia is the prime diagnosis. Always consider the possibility that an ECG abnormality may be related to medical therapy. The patient's history and physical signs will always be more important than the ECG itself.

The ECG may show what is happening to the heart, but as an aid to diagnosis it can do no more than pose questions.

Chapter 6
The physiological basis of the ECG

It is perfectly possible, and not unreasonable, to look at the ECG simply as a tool with which to investigate patients who have symptoms or signs suggesting cardiovascular disease. The ECG can be used in this way with little understanding of the physiological processes involved, and that is why this chapter has been placed at the end of the book. However, it is easier to work out the cause of many ECG abnormalities by thinking in physiological terms, and several ECG abnormalities that are unimportant in that they do not cause symptoms or any impairment of cardiac function are both interesting and important in demonstrating how the heart works.

The cellular basis of the ECG

Contraction of a muscle cell is initiated by an electrical change called depolarisation, and the electrocardiogram (ECG) recorded from the surface of the body results from the depolarisation of all the individual heart muscle cells. The ECG wave form depends on the sequence of the ionic changes that cause depolarisation, and on the way that depolarisation spreads through the heart. When the individual muscle cell is at rest its surface is positively charged and its interior is negatively charged, and the potential difference across the cell membrane is about −90mV. An electrical stimulus can suddenly cause a rapid influx of sodium ions from the extracellular fluid into the cell, so causing the inside of the cell to become positively charged compared with the outside; the transmembrane potential briefly becomes about +30 mV. The initial influx of sodium rapidly ceases but is followed by a slower entry of more sodium ions; at this stage calcium ions also move relatively slowly into the muscle cell and together the entry of these two ions would tend to cause the transmembrane potential to become even more positive. However, the influx of sodium and calcium is balanced by an outflow of potassium ions.

The net electrical result of these later ionic fluxes is that the membrane potential of the muscle cell is held constant at about zero for some 200 ms, and thereafter 'repolarisation' occurs, with a fall of the transmembrane potential to the resting −90mV.

When the surface of one myocardial cell changes its polarity from positive to negative there will be a flux of positive ions in the extracellular fluid away from the adjacent 'resting' cells towards the depolarised cells. This ionic movement triggers depolarisation in the resting cells. Depolarisation therefore spreads outwards like an advancing wave from the cell that was first depolarised. The surface electrocardiogram records this wave of depolarisation; as the myocardial cells are depolarised the ECG records a change of electrical activity at the body surface, but when the myocardial cells are fully depolarised with a constant (zero) membrane potential the ECG returns

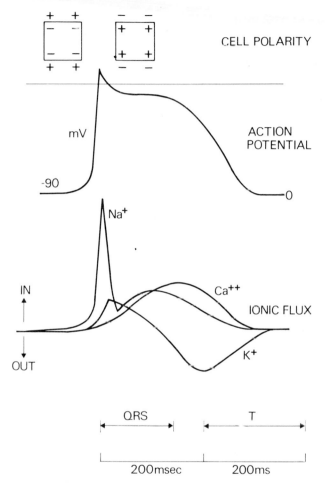

Ionic flux during depolarisation of a single myocardial cell.

to its baseline. During the changes of repolarisation there is a second electrical change at the body surface, and the ECG records a further deflection which is the T wave.

The shape of the P, QRS, and T waves depend on the muscle mass of the atria and ventricles, and upon the speed with which the wave of depolarisation spreads through the heart. The two atria are depolarised together. Their muscle mass is relatively small, and the spread of depolarisation is relatively slow, so the P wave is normally fairly flat and broad.

Following depolarisation of the atrial myocardial cells the ECG returns to baseline. Theoretically an atrial repolarisation wave (an atrial T wave) should be present in the ECG, but in practice this is never seen: the repolarisation process presumably is too diffuse in time to be detected by the standard cardiographic technique. Provided that conduction of depolarisation through the ventricular muscle mass is normal, depolarisation of both ventricles is complete within 120 ms and the ECG complex (the QRS) is narrow. When all the ventricular cells are depolarised the ECG returns to baseline, but as repolarisation occurs the ECG records the ventricular T wave.

Conduction of the depolarisation wave

Depolarisation is normally initiated in the sinoatrial (SA) node, and the depolarisation wave is conducted through the atrial muscle to the AV node. In the AV node conduction is markedly slowed, but from the node originates the only normal electrical connection between the atria and the ventricles, which is the bundle of His. The bundle of His passes from atria to ventricles close to the upper part of the tricuspid valve, and in the inter-ventricular septum divides into left and right branches. The left branch then divides again, into antero-superior, and posterior-inferior branches. Thus three main divisions, or fascicles, of the bundle of His conduct the depolarisation wave rapidly to the Purkinje network and so to the ventricular myocardial cells.

The spread of depolarisation is called conduction, and all cardiac muscle cells possess the property of conductivity. Conduction can occur directly from one muscle cell to another, but this is a relatively slow process. The conduction velocity in atrial myocardial cells is about 1.0 metres per second compared with 0.2 metres per second in the atrioventricular (AV) nodal cells, 4.0 metres per second in the His bundle and ventricular Purkinje cells, and 0.5 metres per second in the ventricular myocardial cells.

Conduction and the electrocardiogram

Conduction of depolarisation can be delayed or 'blocked' anywhere along the pathway from the SA node to the ventricular muscle, and the sites of conduction defects can usually be deduced from the surface ECG.

POSSIBLE SITES FOR CONDUCTION BLOCK

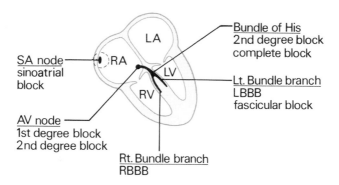

Sino-atrial block. The SA node depolarises normally but the depolarisation wave fails to penetrate the atrium.

SINOATRIAL BLOCK

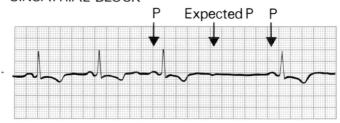

Note: Sinus rhythm for 3 beats then a 'sinus pause'. No P wave is seen but the SA node must have been depolarised because the next P wave appears at the predicted time.

Intra-atrial conduction delay. Because depolarisation spreads through all the atrial muscle conduction defects do not occur but activation of the whole of the atrial myocardium may take longer than normal if the left atrium is hypertrophied. This causes the broad bifid P wave seen in patients with mitral stenosis so long as they remain in sinus rhythm (Ch. 4).

AV node and His bundle block. The PR interval (the period from the onset of the P wave to the first deflection of the QRS complex) measures the time taken for the depolarisation wave to spread from the SA node, through the atria and the AV node and down the His bundle to the inter-ventricular septum, which is the first part of the ventricles to be depolarised. If the PR interval is prolonged, or if the P wave is not followed by a QRS complex, a conduction defect must be present either in the AV node itself or in the His bundle. It is not possible to tell from the surface ECG which of these two sites is involved.

The passage of the depolarisation wave down the His bundle can be detected if an electrode is placed close to the His bundle: this can be done by passing an electrode catheter up a femoral vein and positioning it just through the tricuspid valve. The electrical activity associated with atrial depolarisation recorded in this way is called 'A' rather than 'P', and that associated with ventricular depolarisation is called 'V' rather than 'QRS'. Depolarisation of the His bundle itself is shown as a sharp spike called 'H'.

NORMAL HIS BUNDLE ELECTROGRAM

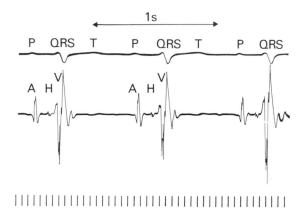

Note: Upper trace shows the usual ECG recorded
from the body surface. The P, QRS and T
waves are broad and flat because the record is
made with a fast paper speed.

The lower trace shows the intracardiac
recording. The 'A' and 'V' waves correspond to
the P and QRS, but have a totally different
appearance.

His bundle depolarisation is shown as a small
spike labelled 'H'.

The A–H interval thus measures the time taken for the depolarisation wave to spread from the SA node to the His bundle, and most of this period is due to AV node delay. In normal subjects the AH interval is between 65 and 115 ms. The H–V interval (normal range 35–55 ms) measures the time for depolarisation to spread from the His bundle to the first part of the interventricular septum.

When each atrial depolarisation is followed by ventricular depolarisation, but atrioventricular conduction is slow, the PR interval on the surface ECG is prolonged and *'first degree block'* is said to be present. This may indicate many varieties of heart disease (for example, it is seen in acute myocardial infarction and acute rheumatic carditis) but of itself it does not impair cardiac function and does not cause symptoms.

1st DEGREE BLOCK

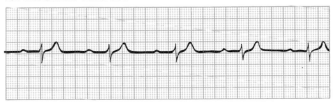

Note: Sinus rhythm.
PR interval is constant at 0.36s.

First degree block commonly occurs in the AV node, and a His bundle electrogram therefore records a prolonged A–H time, but a normal H–V time because conduction in the distal part of the His bundle is normal.

HIS ELECTROGRAM: 1st DEGREE BLOCK

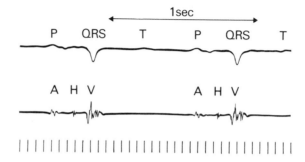

Note: Upper record shows surface ECG.
         Lower record shows His electrogram:
         AH time is prolonged at 150 ms, but the HV
         time is normal at 70 ms.

When atrial depolarisation intermittently fails to induce ventricular depolarisation, *'second degree block'* exists, and this can result from conduction failure anywhere in the AV node or His bundle. There are three varieties:

(a) When most beats are normally conducted but occasionally a P wave is not followed by a QRS. Second degree block of the 'Mobitz Type 2' variety is said to be present. This does not of itself cause symptoms, and its only importance is that it may precede the development of complete block.

2nd DEGREE BLOCK (MOBITZ TYPE II)

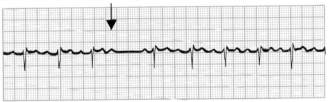

Note: Sinus rhythm with a normal PR interval.
One P wave (arrow) is not followed by QRS.

(b) When the PR interval lengthens progressively with each beat, and then a P wave fails to conduct, the 'Wenckebach phenomenon' is present.

2nd DEGREE BLOCK (WENCKEBACH)

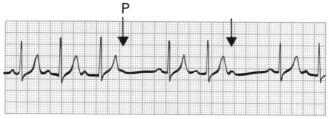

Note: 3 beats with progressively longer PR intervals are followed by a non-conducted P wave (arrow). The next PR interval is short, but this is followed by a longer PR and then another non-conducted beat.

(c) When alternate P waves are not conducted second degree block of the '2:1' type is said to be present.

2nd DEGREE BLOCK (2:1)

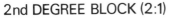
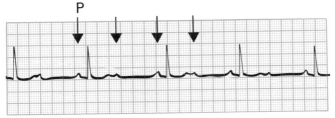

Note: The conducted beats have a normal PR interval, but alternate P waves are not followed by a QRS.

A His bundle electrogram demonstrates the site of second degree block. In the case of 2:1 block this will usually be in the His bundle rather than the AV node, so a normal His spike will be seen but in the non-conducted beats the His spike will not be followed by a V wave.

HIS ELECTROGRAM:2nd DEGREE BLOCK

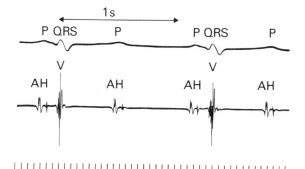

Note: Upper trace shows the surface ECG; as in the other His electrograms the paper speed is fast so the P–QRS–T waves are flattened and spread out. Lower trace shows first a normal A, H, and V but this is followed by an A wave and an H spike with no V wave. The sequence is then repeated.

Second degree block of the Mobitz 2 and Wenckebach types does not cause symptoms. 2:1 block may cause heart failure if the ventricular rate is slow enough.

Third degree, or complete, heart block results either from His bundle disease or from bilateral bundle branch block. When the QRS complex is narrow the rhythm originates within the His bundle itself below the block, but where the QRS is wide ventricular depolarisation originates in the Purkinje system.

COMPLETE (3rd DEGREE) BLOCK

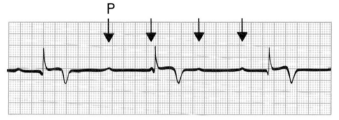

Note: No relationship between P waves (arrowed) and QRS complexes. The QRS complexes are normal; their rate is 30 per minute.

This pattern is commonly seen during an acute inferior myocardial infarction, although the ventricular rate is then usually 50–60 per minute.

COMPLETE HEART BLOCK

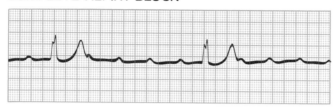

Note: No relationship between P waves and QRS complexes.
Wide QRS with ventricular rate 22 per minute.

Complete heart block does impair cardiac performance: the effect of synchronised atrial contraction is lost and more important, cardiac output falls because of the slow heart rate.

Bundle branch block. When the His bundle conducts normally but one of the bundle branches is blocked, the PR interval is normal but the QRS complex is widened because of late depolarisation of the ventricle normally supplied by the bundle branch which is blocked. Bundle branch block does not significantly impair cardiac function, and of itself is not responsible for any symptoms the patient may have.

Right bundle branch block is characterised by an RSR pattern in lead V_1.

RIGHT BUNDLE BRANCH BLOCK

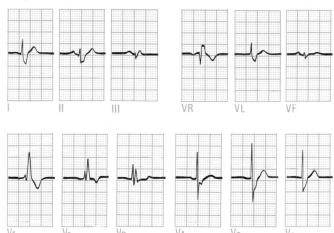

Note: Sinus rhythm with a normal PR interval.
Right axis deviation.
RSR pattern in V_1; the dominant R wave is characteristic of RBBB and does not indicate RV hypertrophy.
Wide and slurred S wave in V_6.

Left bundle branch block is characterised by a loss of the septal Q wave and notching of the QRS complex in lead V_6.

LEFT BUNDLE BRANCH BLOCK

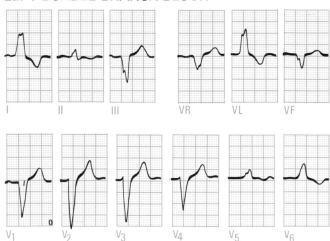

V leads at ½ sensitivity

Note: Sinus rhythm.

Broad QRS with notch in the R wave in leads I, III, VL, VF and V_5. Remember that inverted T waves are associated with bundle branch block and have no other significance.

If a bundle branch block is associated with first degree block it is likely that the remaining bundle branch is diseased, and that bilateral bundle branch block (causing third degree block) is imminent.

1st DEGREE BLOCK AND BUNDLE BRANCH BLOCK

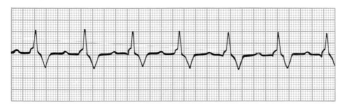

Note: Sinus rhythm.
        PR interval 0.28 s (first degree block).
        Broad QRS and inverted T waves indicate bundle branch block, but in a single monitoring lead such as this it is not possible to say which bundle branch is blocked.

Fascicular block. The right bundle branch is a single structure but the left bundle divides into two branches or fascicles. Depolarisation spreads into the left ventricle through these fascicles, and the average of these two directions of depolarisation as seen from the front is called the frontal plane vector or cardiac axis.

THE NORMAL CARDIAC AXIS

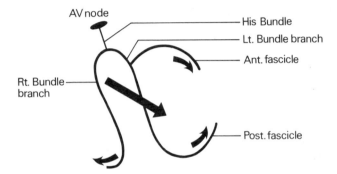

Note: Small arrows show the direction of spread of depolarisation through the main branches of the His bundle. Broad arrow shows the average direction of spread of depolarisation in these three branches, as seen from the front. This is the 'cardiac axis'.

Failure of conduction in the antero superior branch of the left bundle (left anterior fascicular block or 'left anterior hemiblock') means that the left ventricle has to be depolarised through the posterior fascicle. The average direction of depolarisation, the cardiac axis, therefore swings upwards and causes left axis deviation.

LEFT ANTERIOR HEMIBLOCK

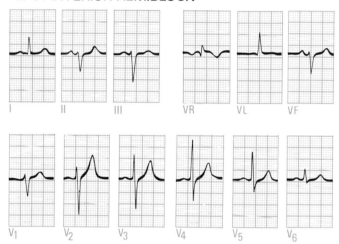

Note: Sinus rhythm with a normal PR interval. The average direction of depolarisation in the standard leads is mainly towards I and VL, and away from both II and III which show predominant S waves. This is left axis deviation.

Failure of conduction in the posterior inferior fascicle (left posterior hemiblock) causes the cardiac axis to swing to the right and this is shown by a deep S wave in lead I. This is seen much less often than left anterior hemiblock.

The combination of right bundle branch block and left anterior hemiblock indicates disease of two of the three main ventricular conducting pathways. This is an example of 'bifascicular' block.

BIFASCICULAR BLOCK

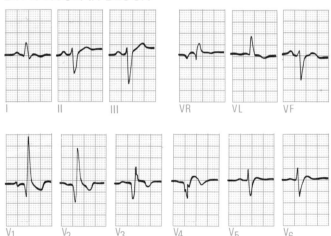

Note: Sinus rhythm with a normal PR interval.
Left axis deviation.
RSR pattern in V_1 and deep S in V_6 show RBBB.

Rhythms resulting from cardiac automaticity

Myocardial cells are only depolarised when they are stimulated, but the cells of the sinoatrial node, those around the atrioventricular node (the 'junctional' cells) and the cells of the conducting pathways all possess the property of spontaneous depolarisation or 'automaticity'. The transmembrane potential wave form of these cells is quite different from that of the myocardial cells: there is a slow upward drift during diastole, and when it reaches a critical threshold, depolarisation occurs.

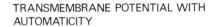

TRANSMEMBRANE POTENTIAL WITH AUTOMATICITY

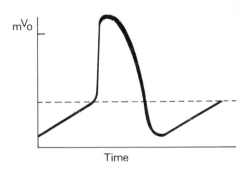

This automatic depolarisation is quite regular, although it can be influenced by physiological and pharmacological factors: the classic example of this is 'sinus arrhythmia', where SA node activity is affected by the waxing and waning influence of the vagus nerve.

SINUS ARRHYTHMIA

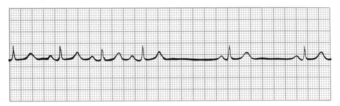

Note: Although the R–R interval varies markedly, the shape of the P waves and the duration of the PR intervals are constant. The irregularity in the rate of QRS complexes must therefore be due to sinus arrhythmia.

Loss of sino atrial node activity causes 'sinus arrest', a rhythm common in the sick sinus syndrome. The ECG abnormality is differentiated from sinoatrial block because the next P wave does not appear until after 2 (or 3) normal intervals.

SINUS ARREST

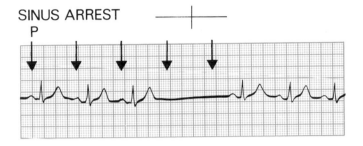

Note: Sinus rhythm.

After 3 beats there is a 'sinus pause' with no P wave.

Arrows mark where the next two P waves should have been.

Sinus rhythm is then restored, but the cycle has been reset.

The automaticity of any part of the heart is suppressed by the arrival of a depolarisation wave, and the heart rate is therefore controlled by the region with the highest automatic depolarisation frequency. Normally the SA node controls the heart because it has the highest frequency of discharge, but if for any reason this fails the region with the next highest intrinsic depolarisation frequency will emerge as the pacemaker and set up an 'escape' rhythm. The atria and the junctional region have automatic depolarisation frequencies of about 50 per minute, compared with the normal SA node rate of 60 or 70 per minute. If both the SA node and the junctional region fail to depolarise, a ventricular focus may emerge, with a rate of 30—40 per minute; this is seen classically in complete heart block where although SA node automaticity is normal, the impulse is not conducted to the ventricles.

Escape beats may be single, or may form sustained rhythms. They have the same ECG appearance as the corresponding extrasystoles, which of course appear early rather than late.

JUNCTIONAL ESCAPE BEAT

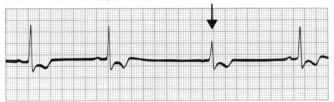

Note: After 2 sinus beats there is no P wave.
After an interval there is a narrow QRS
complex with the same configuration as that of
the sinus beats, but without a preceding P
wave. This is a junctional beat. Sinus rhythm
then reappears.

JUNCTIONAL ESCAPE RHYTHM

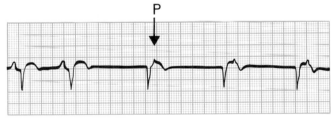

Note: 2 sinus beats are followed by an interval with
no P waves.
A junctional rhythm then emerges (QRS
complexes the same as in sinus rhythm).
A P wave can be seen as a hump on the T wave
of the junctional beats: the atria have been
depolarised retrogradely.

JUNCTIONAL RHYTHM

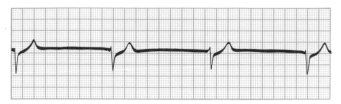

Note: No P waves.
Narrow QRS complexes and normal T waves.

VENTRICULAR ESCAPE BEAT

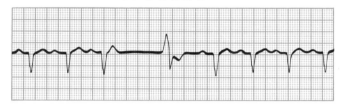

Note: 3 sinus beats are followed by a pause. There is
a single ventricular beat with a wide QRS and
an inverted T wave. Sinus rhythm is then
restored.

If the intrinsic frequency of depolarisation of atrial,
junctional, or ventricular conducting tissue is
increased, an abnormal rhythm may occur: this
phenomenon is called 'enhanced automaticity'. The
most common example of a sustained rhythm due to
enhanced automaticity is 'accelerated idioventricular
rhythm' which is common after acute myocardial

infarction. The ECG appearances resemble a slow
ventricular tachycardia, and this is the old fashioned
name for this condition. This rhythm causes no
symptoms and should not be treated.

ACCELERATED IDIOVENTRICULAR RHYTHM

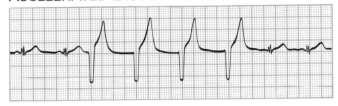

Note: After 2 sinus beats there are 4 beats of
           ventricular origin with a rate of 75 per minute.
           Sinus rhythm is then restored.

An accelerated idionodal rhythm may appear to
'overtake' P waves when the enhanced junctional
automatic rate approximates to that of the SA node.

ACCELERATED IDIONODAL RHYTHM

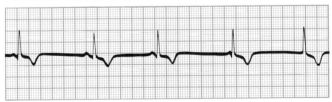

Note: After 3 sinus beats the sinus rate slows
           slightly.
           A nodal rhythm appears and 'overtakes' the P
           waves.

Enhanced automaticity is also thought to be the mechanism of some non-paroxysmal tachycardias, particularly those due to digitalis intoxication.

Abnormalities of cardiac rhythm due to re-entry

Normal conduction involves the uniform spread of the depolarisation wave front in a constant direction. Should the direction of depolarisation be reversed in some part of the heart it is possible for a circular or 're-entry' pathway to be set up round which depolarisation reverberates, causing a tachycardia. The anatomical requirement is branching and rejoining of a conduction pathway. Normally conduction is anterograde (forward) in both limbs of this pathway, but if conduction in one limb is slower than in the other an anterograde impulse may pass normally down one but be blocked in the other. Where the pathways rejoin the depolarisation wave can spread retrogradely (backwards) up the abnormal branch, and if it should arrive at a time when that pathway is no longer refractory to conduction, it can pass right round the circuit and reactivate it. Once established this circuitous spread of depolarisation may continue.

RE ENTRY MECHANISM OF TACHYCARDIAS

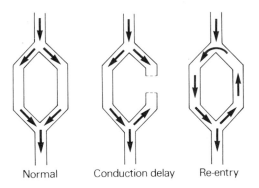

Normal   Conduction delay   Re-entry

   The classical — though not the most common —
example of this is the Wolff-Parkinson-White (WPW)
syndrome (See Ch. 2).
   Where the anatomical circuit is relatively large, (as
in the WPW syndrome) 'macro-re-entry' is said to
occur. Macro-re-entry circuits can also occur within
the atrial and ventricular myocardium, and are
responsible for paroxysmal atrial flutter, atrial
fibrillation, and ventricular tachycardia.

ATRIAL FLUTTER WITH CAROTID SINUS PRESSURE (CSP)

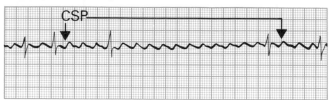

Note: Atrial flutter with 2:1 block. Carotid sinus
pressure completely suppresses AV
conduction, and there is no QRS complex for 3
seconds.

In atrial fibrillation, 'flutter-like' waves sometimes
appear intermittently, and these depend on re-entry
through circuits of varying lengths.
'Flutter-fibrillation' behaves clinically like atrial
fibrillation.

ATRIAL FIBRILLATION

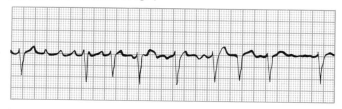

Note: Atrial fibrillation with varying QRS rate but
constant QRS configuration.
Initially 'flutter' waves are present, but later
these are replaced by the typical chaotic
baseline of fibrillation.

In ventricular tachycardia the broad QRS complexes are of a constant configuration and are fairly regular if the re-entry pathway is constant.

VENTRICULAR TACHYCARDIA

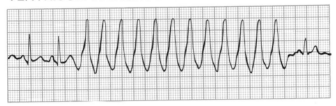

Note: 2 sinus beats are followed by ventricular tachycardia at 150 per minute. The complexes are regular with little variation in shape. Sinus rhythm is then restored.

However, the re-entry path often varies slightly causing variation in the QRS shape and some irregularity in its timing. This is seen in the most extreme form in the 'Torsade de Pointes' variety of ventricular tachycardia.

VENTRICULAR TACHYCARDIA

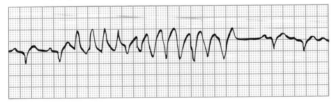

Note: 2 sinus beats are followed by ventricular tachycardia. The complexes initially point upwards but then become inverted, and the QRS rate is variable.

Junctional or AV nodal tachycardia (sometimes inappropriately called 'supra-ventricular tachycardia') is also due to re-entry, but here 'micro-re-entry' occurs through tracts within the AV node itself.

JUNCTIONAL TACHYCARDIA

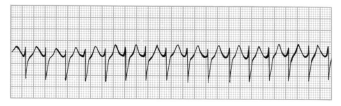

Note: No P waves can be seen. The QRS complexes are narrow and completely regular at 160 per minute.

Except for the pre-excitation syndromes, there is no certain way of differentiating from the surface ECG a tachycardia due to enhanced automaticity from one due to re-entry. In general, however, tachycardias that follow extrasystoles, or those that can be initiated or inhibited by appropriately timed intracardiac pacing impulses, are likely to be due to re-entry.

ATRIAL TACHYCARDIA

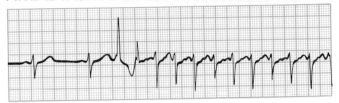

Note: After 2 sinus beats there is one ventricular
extrasystole and a narrow complex which is
probably supraventricular.
Atrial tachycardia is induced; P waves are
visible at the end of the T wave of the
preceding beat.

JUNCTIONAL TACHYCARDIA

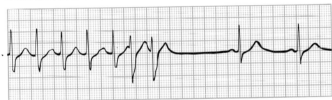

Note: 5 beats of junctional tachycardia at 150 per
minute are followed by 2 ventricular
extrasystoles. These interrupt the tachycardia
and sinus rhythm is restored.

The differentiation between the two mechanisms is
at present only of theoretical importance.

Conclusions

The ECG is easy to understand, and most of its abnormalities are amenable to reason. Like everything in biology and medicine there are quite marked variations both in the ECGs of normal subjects and in the ECG patterns that accompany specific diseases, and it is these variations that sometimes make the ECG seem difficult. These variations will be recognised with practice, and there is no substitute for reporting large numbers of ECGs, whether these be normal or abnormal.

However, the key to the ECG is to use it as an adjunct to the history and physical examination. When in doubt it is better to depend on these than on the ECG, and it is always the patient who should be treated, not the ECG.

Index